Acclaim for Pauline W. Chen's

FINAL EXAM

"[*Final Exam* is] a series of thoughtful, moving essays. . . . [Chen's] most hopeful argument is herself: a doctor open to confronting her own fears and doubts, and willing to prepare her patients for the final exam."
                                        —*The New York Times*

"In restrained but impassioned prose, Chen brings home to us the gritty truths that doctors confront daily."   —*Elle*

"Compassionate, compelling."   —*People*

"An affecting, convincing look at the questions of death from a physician's point of view—presented with honesty."   —*Deseret News* (Salt Lake City)

"Chen writes with tenderness and clarity, as if sharing her most intimate thoughts and concerns with a close friend . . . . Chen's deep compassion and humanity shine in this narrative. Her devotion to patients as well as her honesty about life and death issues make this a compelling read."
                                        Rocky Mountain News

"Chen uses words with a surgeon's precision, courageously confronting difficult subject matter with stunning results. She aces this 'Final Exam.'"   —*New York Post*

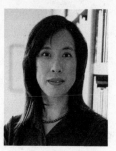

Pauline W. Chen

FINAL EXAM

Pauline W. Chen attended Harvard University and the
Feinberg School of Medicine at Northwestern University
and completed her surgical training at Yale University, the National Cancer Institute (National Institutes
of Health), and UCLA, where she was most recently a
member of the faculty. In 1999, she was named the
UCLA Outstanding Physician of the Year. Dr. Chen's first
nationally published piece, "Dead Enough? The Paradox of Brain Death," appeared in *The Virginia Quarterly
Review* and was a finalist for a 2006 National Magazine
Award. She is also the 2005 cowinner of the Staige D.
Blackford Prize for Nonfiction and was a finalist for the
2002 James Kirkwood Prize in Creative Writing. She
lives near Boston with her husband and children.

Dr. Pauline Chen is available for lectures and readings.
For information regarding her availability, please visit
www.knopfspeakersbureau.com or call 212-572-2013.

FINAL EXAM

A
Surgeon's Reflections
on Mortality

PAULINE W. CHEN

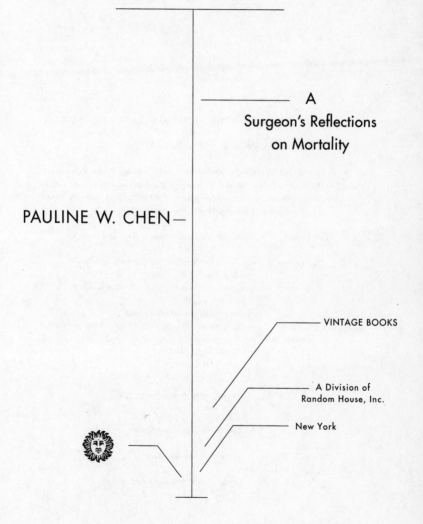

VINTAGE BOOKS

A Division of
Random House, Inc.

New York

FIRST VINTAGE BOOKS EDITION, JANUARY 2008

Copyright © 2007 by Pauline W. Chen

All rights reserved. Published in the United States by Vintage Books, a division of
Random House, Inc., New York, and in Canada by Random House of Canada Limited,
Toronto. Originally published in hardcover in the United States by Alfred A. Knopf,
a division of Random House, Inc., New York, in 2007.

Vintage and colophon are registered trademarks of Random House, Inc.

The Library of Congress has cataloged the Knopf edition as follows:
Chen, Pauline W., 1964–
Final exam : a surgeon's reflections on mortality / Pauline W. Chen.
p. cm.
Includes bibliographical references.
1. Chen, Pauline W., 1964– 2. Surgeons—Biography. 3. Death—Moral and ethical
aspects. 4. Terminal care—moral and ethical aspects. I. Title.
RD27.35.C47A3 2007
617.092—dc22
[B] 2006049361

Vintage ISBN: 978-0-307-27537-0

Author photograph © Joanne Chan
Book design by Soonyoung Kwon

www.vintagebooks.com

Printed in the United States of America
10 9 8 7 6 5 4 3 2

To my father and mother for the past,
to Natalie and Isabelle for the future,
and to Woody for the here and now.

Note to the Reader

The narratives in this book are true. A few of the subjects—
Erika, Celia, Susan, Hasan, Dorinne, and my family members—
have permitted me to use their real names. In all the other
narratives, I have changed the names and the identifying details
in order to maintain confidentiality.

CONTENTS

III. REAPPRAISAL

INTRODUCTION

Erika's voice on the other end of the line has the same soprano clarity I remember from college. It has been nearly twenty years—and between us, two completed residencies, two weddings, and four children—since our last conversation, but my college roommate and I are talking again, helped in part by the breezy missives of the Internet. Earlier that afternoon I received an e-mail from Erika briefly telling me that her father, Dr. Schillinger, a clinical psychologist, had just died. *It's made me want to reconnect with the past,* she wrote.

I remember Erika's father. One afternoon when her parents were visiting, Erika put a Tommy Dorsey record on our feeble dorm room sound system. I watched Dr. Schillinger in his navy cardigan and low-perched reading glasses rise from our red vinyl couch, grab Erika's right hand, and twirl her to the music. His Hitchcockesque silhouette became weightless, and he danced in a way that I believed impossible for someone's parent.

On the phone Erika tells me that last year her father was diagnosed with metastatic gastric cancer. He tried a few rounds of chemotherapy but developed pulmonary fibrosis, a stiffening of the lungs that slowly suffocates. Bed-bound and weakened by the slightest exertion, Dr. Schillinger persisted in crooning to Erika's eight-month-old daughter, making her shimmy as he sang. By the end of each line the alarm on his blood oxygenation monitor would cry out, but Dr. Schillinger, ignoring the electronic warnings and Erika's pleas to stop, would warble on.

When the struggle to breathe finally became unbearable, Dr. Schillinger signaled to his daughter: he wanted only to be comfortable. Despite his terminal diagnosis, Dr. Schillinger's doctors had made no provisions for this moment. Instead, in his last hours Dr. Schillinger had to look to Erika, his physician daughter, for guidance. None of his doctors was even present, and it was Erika who had to ask for morphine, knowing that the drug would both alleviate her father's suffering and suppress his drive to breathe.

Talking to me a month after, Erika weeps, remembering the responsibility of the moment. "Do you know how many times 'death' was mentioned during those last few months?" she asks me. I cannot begin to guess; anyone with some medical training could have seen that Dr. Schillinger was a terminal patient.

"Once," she says, that crystalline voice faltering. "A doctor discussed dying once with us. Otherwise, all anyone ever talked about was treating my father." Erika pauses and then asks me, "Why are we so bad at taking care of the dying?"

Twenty years ago when I was applying to medical school, I believed I was going to save lives. Like the heroic doctors of my imagination, I would spend my days in triumphant face-offs with death and watch the parade of saved patients return to my office full of life, smiles, and back-slapping gratitude. What I did not count on was how much death would be a part of my work.

In a profession made attractive by the power to cure, it is rare to find the young medical student who dreams of caring for terminal patients. But in a society where more than 90 percent of us will die from a prolonged illness, physicians have become the final guardians of life, charged with shepherding the terminally ill and their families through the intricacies of the end. Most patients and their families fully expect physicians to be able to comfort and provide that support. For doctors, this care at the end of life is, as this book's title implies, our final exam.

Unfortunately, few doctors are up to the task.

Like most of my colleagues, I came into medicine poorly equipped to deal with terminal patients. I had little experience with the dying beforehand and like many physicians harbored a profound aversion to death. However, during almost fifteen years of school and training, I faced death over and over again. And I learned from many of my teachers and colleagues to suspend or suppress any shared human feelings for my dying patients, as if doing so would make me a better doctor. These lessons in denial and depersonalization began as early as my first encounter with death in the gross anatomy dissection lab and were reinforced during the chaos of residency training and practice.

As I learned and eventually even mimicked these coping mechanisms, I found myself wrestling with disturbing inconsistencies that only multiplied over time. There was a dying friend I could not call, a young patient's tortured death that I could not forget, and even the sense of shared humanity with a corpse that I could not cast aside when I was asked to saw her pelvis in two. These small but powerful moments, magnified every time I encountered death, would finally give me insight into how my own fears and trained responses had, in the end, incapacitated me. In acknowledging the painful consequences and paradoxes of my behavior, I began to extricate myself from those learned responses. Amid the pain of losing patients, I learned that I might be able to do something greater than cure. I could provide comfort to my patients and their families and in turn open myself to receive some of their greatest lessons.

Final Exam: A Surgeon's Reflections on Mortality is a compilation of my experiences dealing with death. It weaves personal narratives from fifteen years of clinical experience with reflections on some of the broader issues in medical education and end-of-life care. The first section, "Principles," focuses on the earliest lessons in medical school regarding death—the cadaver dissection, the first resuscitation, the first pronouncement of death. These earliest experiences pit the neophyte medical student and intern against some of the most difficult—some would call them terrifying—experiences in clinical medicine, often without the benefit of much psychological or emotional preparation. The lessons young doctors draw from these experiences then become the foundations of their future practices.

The second section, "Practice," delves into the heart of clinical work, revealing how our professional responses not only manifest but also perpetuate themselves. There is an essential paradox in medicine: a profession premised on caring for the ill also systematically depersonalizes dying. However, when viewed from within the daily rhythms of clinical work, there is an internally coherent logic. What seems inhumane or cruel—evading difficult patient conversations, ramping up treatment in terminal diseases—can be entirely rational to the foot soldiers in the clinical trenches. And that logic makes change, at least for the practicing resident, seem nearly impossible.

The final section, "Reappraisal," explores how change is in fact possible. From the microcosm of a single doctor's practice to the medical profession as a whole, there have been small but hopeful transformations in how doctors approach end-of-life care. And these changes have been the result of more than just critical appraisals of our professional training and institutions; they have required recognizing our own mortality and a shared humanity with our patients.

Whether we are physicians or not, facing that mortality in ourselves is perhaps the most difficult task of all. As Freud wrote, "[I]n the unconscious every one of us is convinced of his own immortality." It is nearly impossible as we go about our daily duties to talk about our lives as finite. Nonetheless, it is only by taking on these discussions that we can ensure our patients—and our loved ones—a good death, however each person may define that. Freud went on to say:

> We remember the old saying: *Si vis pacem, para bellum.* If you desire peace, prepare for war. It would be timely thus to paraphrase it: *Si vis vitam, para mortem.* If you would endure life, be prepared for death.

Preparing for death may be the most difficult exam of all, but it is the one that will, finally, free us to live.

I

PRINCIPLES

Chapter 1

RESURRECTIONIST

My very first patient had been dead for over a year before I laid hands on her.

It was the mid-1980s, and I had at last made the transition from premedical to full-fledged medical student. That late summer from the window of my dormitory room, I could see the vastness of Lake Michigan dotted with sailboats and the grunting, glistening runners loping along its Chicago shores. Despite this placid view, I rarely looked out my window. I was far too preoccupied with what lay ahead: my classmates and I were about to begin the dissection of a human cadaver.

Prior to that September, the only time I had seen a

dead person was at the funeral of my Agong, my maternal grandfather. Agong had grown up on a farm in the backwaters of Taiwan at the turn of the last century. He barely finished high school, but by the time he was middle-aged, Agong owned a jewelry store in one of Taipei's most fashionable districts and had raised five college-educated children. While he grew up speaking Taiwanese, Agong had taught himself Mandarin Chinese and Japanese, languages and dialects as different as German, English, and French.

Agong loved my mother, his firstborn child, and lavished her with that gift of nearly blind parental adoration. As *her* firstborn child, I was in a special position to receive some of those rays of love. Unfortunately though, with my American upbringing I understood Taiwanese but spoke only "Chinglish," a pidgin amalgamation of English and Mandarin Chinese. Moreover, Agong and I had been separated by half a world until he moved permanently to the United States when I was in high school. So while I loved my grandfather, our relationship always remained rather formal.

Agong died in the fall of my sophomore year in college. One weekend, my parents mentioned to me on the phone that he was doing worse and might possibly "not make it." A week later they called again to tell me that he had passed away.

My mother was grief-stricken. She became consumed by guilt and remorse, feelings that I would later learn often plague relatives of the recently dead. For my part, while I did mourn Agong's death, I was unsure how to cope with this phase of life or with my mother's overwhelming grief. I had not been witness to his actual dying, and seeing my grandfather alive during one visit and lying dead in a casket the next made his death unreal to me. The funeral was not particularly long, but the parade of mourners dressed in black and my own uneasy feelings seemed to last forever.

I was surprised by how *un*-lifelike Agong looked lying in the casket. Despite all the efforts of the mortician, the figure in the coffin simply looked like a model of Agong, like a wax figure from Madame Tussauds's famous museum. His face and body as I had known them were gone. Even his nose, famous in our family for its Jimmy Durante profile, had changed; the nostrils looked less fleshy and even droopy, like a once majestic sail that had lost its wind.

The fact that even the professionals with all their makeup and tricks could not re-create my grandfather's likeness only served to emphasize that he was really dead and gone from our lives. That funeral, the telephone call from my parents announcing my grandfather's passing, and the memories of my mother's grieving were the most direct experiences with death that I had prior to medical school.

The majority of my 170 medical school classmates were no more experienced than I, and our first real exposure to death would be that semester in the human anatomy course. While one student had worked in a hospital morgue during college and another had worked in an Illinois meatpacking plant (subsequently becoming a strict vegetarian), those two classmates were the rare exception. Instead, the summer before starting medical school most of us privately dreaded and fretted about dissecting a human being.

During my medical school orientation week, I was finally able to share my dissection fears with others who harbored the same uneasiness. Anatomy quickly became a major topic of discussion at social events. The classmate who had worked in a morgue was a prime source of information for the rest of us. I kept wondering if the cadavers looked alive or like wax figures. I secretly hoped that they would look at least as unreal as my grandfather had, believing that the less they looked like the living, the easier dissecting would be. We asked the second-year medical students about their experience the previous year. "Wear your old T-shirts and jeans," they said, sipping their drinks nonchalantly at receptions for the new initiates. "You'll want to throw out those clothes at the end of the semester because they'll just reek." Holding on to their words, I replayed their cavalier responses in my mind. What smell would cling to our clothes? Death?

From the moment I had begun contemplating this career path some fifteen years earlier, I knew that I would want to use my profession to help people. Most of my classmates were no different. We were an odd group, idealistic but intensely obsessive and competitive enough to have survived the grueling premedical curriculum. While a few of us might have harbored goals of financial security or visions of a certain lifestyle, we were for the most part determined to learn how to save lives.

What many of us did not realize was that despite those dreams, our profession would require us to live among the dying. Death, more than life, would become the constant in our lives.

The dissection of the human body had fascinated me since I was seven years old. I had some idea back then that I might want to become a doctor. At the time my Agong had just been diagnosed with a brain tumor, and my mother took my younger sister and me back to Taiwan for the summer to be with him. The diagnosis, the operation, and the neurologic deficits resulting from the removal of a part of my grandfather's brain would eventually color the rest of my grandparents' lives together. Nonetheless, at the time I was enthralled by the way his neurosurgeon comforted my grandmother and family. He was a big, bald Taiwanese man, with a round face, hands like bear paws, and a demeanor that was at once humble and confident. When he came out to the waiting room to an audience of anxious family members, his words—"I got it all out"—fell on us like a great light from the heavens. That experience convinced me that medicine was the work of gods.

An aunt who was in medical school at the time heard about my interest and offered to take me to her anatomy lab. I was fascinated by the idea that there might be secrets about life and death lurking there. At that age I already had come to believe that dissection was the greatest event that separated physicians from the rest of us. To be able to stomach such an experience, I thought, would prove my mettle, and to sneak a peek into the inner workings of a body—a dead body, no less—would put me in a league beyond any other second-grader I knew. My parents, however, quickly vetoed the idea, fearing that such a close-up and possibly gruesome experience might scar me permanently.

Like all initiation rites, the dissection of the human cadaver poses several obstacles to the neophyte. First, the new medical student has to memorize a vast array of anatomical facts. Such rote memorization can be mind-numbingly dull, and the overwhelming amount of information makes the task seem Sisyphean. One of my college mentors, a brilliant psychiatrist and anthropologist, counseled me before I started. He had completed medical school some twenty years earlier. "It's like memorizing a telephone book," he said. "You just have to get through it."

Memorization, however, is probably the easiest obstacle to surmount, and it has until recently been the only focus of medical schools. The more difficult, and often unspoken, obstacle for medical students is accepting death and the violation of the human body. In the human anatomy course, cadavers are laid before fledgling physicians, and the familiarity of their form reminds us that each lived lives not unlike our own. For those of us who wince from simple paper cuts, running a scalpel against skin and definitively dividing the essential structures that once powered a fellow human are acts that require a leap of faith. While all premedical students fully expect to perform a human cadaver dissection in medical school, the expectation hardly tempers the brutal reality.

Aspiring physicians face death directly in the form of the cadaver. And then they tear it apart. Each detail of the cadaver—every bone, nerve, blood vessel, and muscle—passes from the world of the unknown into the realm of the familiar. Every cavity is probed, every groove explored, and every crevice pulled apart. In knowing the cadaver in such intimate detail, we believe that we are acquiring the knowledge to overcome death.

To complete the initiation rite successfully, however, we need to learn to separate our emotional self from our scientific self; we must view this dead human body not as "one of us" but as "one of them," a medical case to be understood but not embraced. This ability to distance the self, I was to learn later, would be called upon again and again in my medical training. It was as if such separation would provide me with a greater sense of objectivity, a modicum of strength, and thus an enhanced ability to care for my patients. But this first lesson in disengaging from the personal was the most radical: it required suppressing the fundamental and very human fear of death.

. . .

My medical school, not entirely unaware of the anxiety we harbored, did make some attempts to lessen the impact of working with a cadaver. We spent a week in lectures preparing for the first day of dissection. While none of these lectures directly addressed our mounting anxieties, they did give us the tools we needed to begin to detach ourselves emotionally from the experience. One of our first anatomic lessons was on vocabulary used to describe the body. These words, so different from our usual descriptive terms, would serve as directions on the map of the human body. We learned the difference between "distal" and "proximal," "abduct" and "adduct," "transverse" and "sagittal." We learned that "left" and "right" no longer referred to our left and right but to the patient's.

The day before our first dissection lab, we toured the laboratory facilities. There were eleven rooms connected by a long hallway, and each room had four large stone lab benches with sinks and enough workspace for four students. A large enclosed cavity within the lab benches held a sliding metal bed not unlike the metal beds used by coroners or pathologists. These cavities would be where our cadavers would be stored. We would spend every weekday afternoon for the next twelve weeks in these rooms, and all of us, either in small groups or alone, would spend many of our free hours there trying to memorize the minutiae from each cadaver.

Formaldehyde, the preservative used for cadavers, has an unmistakable odor—sharp, rancid, piercing—like the olfactory version of a high-pitched shriek. The faint smell of formaldehyde present in each of the eleven rooms was left over from years past, as the cadavers for our class had not yet arrived. Over the years the smell had managed to work its way into the rooms' marble and concrete, lingering and reminding us of our place in the school's history.

Our professor was not the wizened sage I had always envisioned would take me through this rite. Instead, he was just a few years out from his own graduate work in physical anthropology and anatomy. His youth and strong Hoosier twang demystified the whole ritual and made many of us more relaxed. He informed us of the overwhelming power of the scent of formaldehyde and reminded us that the smell would permeate our gloved hands, clothes, and hair. Indeed, I would soon discover that it would be strange eating with my hands that semester. While tasting some chicken wings at a reception later that fall, I realized that the smell of the cadavers from my fingers was mingling with the taste of barbecued chicken in my mouth. "Lemon dishwashing detergent helps get rid of the smell," our professor advised us the afternoon before we were to embark on our dissections. That night each of us pulled out clothes that we were willing to toss at the end of three months—frayed jeans, "borrowed" hospital scrubs, and T-shirts with high school emblems—and there was a run on lemon dishwashing detergent at the local grocery stores.

The next afternoon an intensified odor assaulted each of us as we entered the labs; overnight, the laboratory technicians had placed fresh cadavers in their respective stone enclaves. For that afternoon's work I had replaced my contact lenses, susceptible to the fumes of formaldehyde, with my chunky glasses, and I remember being mildly surprised by how many of my fellow classmates were as blind as I. All of us had also carefully put on thin yellow paper masks, more to blunt the penetrating

formaldehyde than to protect ourselves from any bio-
hazards. Over the weeks, as we became more absorbed in
our work, we eventually neglected to wear these flimsy
barriers. Some of us even occasionally forgot to put on our
gloves.

The class was divided alphabetically into groups of
four students, and each group was assigned to a cadaver.
These groupings were used over and over again during the
next two years whenever our education required more intimate instruction. With the same three classmates, we
clumsily attempted to draw blood, learned to do pelvic
exams, and performed our first rectal exams on patients.
Most notably, however, we dissected together in anatomy lab.

I worked with three other women. Mary was from
California, the daughter of a family practitioner and the
middle child in a large Irish-Italian Catholic family. She
was preternaturally calm, a characteristic that would give
her an outstanding bedside manner, and she eventually
followed in her father's footsteps. Peg was from Chicago.
She was the most reticent of the four but made up for her
shyness with a generous spirit and a sharp, dry wit that
helped give the rest of us perspective during more difficult
times. She later became a pediatrician. The third woman,
Lara, was the youngest and the most boisterous of the four
of us. The daughter of immigrants, she was born and raised
in Chicago and now practices pediatrics in that city. I
was from New England and set at the time on becoming a
psychiatrist or geriatrician and pursuing an academic
career in medical anthropology. However, as gruesome as
it all seemed to me that first week, the experience of
the cadaver dissection—the concise and efficient beauty
of human anatomy, the pleasure of using my hands as
an extension of my mind, and the spirit of teamwork—

became the foundation of my decision to become a surgeon.

On that first day I unlatched the door on the side of our stone lab bench and gently slid the metal bed out of the inner compartment. All the cadavers were sheathed in white plastic body bags. Some bags were large; others were smaller. There was no question, however, given the frozen forms, what was within these zippered shrouds. Several provisions had been made by the medical school to decrease the shock of starting our work. The lab technicians had placed all the bodies facedown so that we could see only the back of their head. We started our daily dissections with the arms and legs, and our cadavers' faces were kept covered until the final two weeks of the course. Those who organized our anatomy course believed that such a progression would be a gentler introduction to working on a dead human being.

We learned anatomic principles, dissection techniques, and ways to hold the dissecting instruments with greater precision. We learned that in medicine, "tweezers" were called "forceps," and those who fancied a future career in surgery used the more specialized jargon, "pickups." We learned to change blades efficiently on a scalpel without ever touching the blade's sharp edge, to hold the scalpel like a pencil for finer work, and to grasp it with the tips of four fingers and the thumb apposed, as if holding a violin bow, for more dramatic slices and cuts. We began to manipulate scissors with the thumb and fourth finger, as surgeons do, not the thumb and index finger as we had once learned in nursery school. "Using the fourth finger allows the index finger to rest on the joint of the scissors and gives greater control," stated one of the teaching assistants, a fourth-year medical student planning on a surgical career. Hairdressers everywhere, I would later note, hold scissors in a similar fashion.

The only information that we had on our cadavers was a card attached to the bag indicating their gender and approximate age at death. My cadaver was a woman who had died at seventy-two. Other than those two pieces of information, there was nothing else: no name, no address, no story. It was unsettling to be presented with so little history, and it became more so as we allowed ourselves to become intimately familiar with every detail of these bodies. My lab partners and I would know our cadaver's body better than any patient we would ever take care of; yet in her book of life, we were to begin with the epilogue and attempt to read backward.

Despite all the precautions taken by my medical school, my cadaver hardly remained an impersonal corpse with anonymous extremities. I remember unzipping the white bag that held her and being surprised by her thin arms. Her fingers were long and slender, with delicate, pointed tips; her nails had been filed into fine ovals and painted with coral nail polish. It was probably time for another manicure, as just above her neatly maintained cuticles were slender little half-moons of bare pink nail. While the skin around her forearm seemed to wrap tightly around her muscles, the skin on her upper arm was looser. It was wrinkled and hardened, like old leather. I figured that the hardening must have been from the time spent in a vat of formaldehyde.

My lab partners and I took scalpels to the skin of our cadaver, making long incisions along the length of the hand and forearm. In so interrupting the tension of the skin, we released the dermal tissue and muscles from their epidermal cocoons. We then gently stripped and separated that tissue with fine scissors and forceps, traveling along the axes of the vessels and nerves. Moving our cadaver's arm, now free of any skin covering or sinewy attachments, we saw the muscles function with each action and wondered how much more animated they might have been in life.

Aspects of that life were apparent from our cadaver's slender arms. She had loved the sun; the tanned background of her skin betrayed the jewelry that had once adorned her. On her left fourth finger I could see the white imprint of a wedding band. On her wrist I could make out the pale outline of a watch, probably one of those fine old-lady watches with the delicate chain across the latch for security. As we dissected into her hand, encountering the small muscles—flexor pollicis longus, abductor pollicis brevis—I could imagine how each of these bundles of tissue once worked in her hands. The pink flesh, now a grayish red in death, would have contracted, each fiber shortening and swelling with the exertion, the muscle strands pulling on their attachments to her fingers, flexing the fingers around the hand of her husband or the brush she held to her hair.

Trying to memorize the Latin names with no intrinsic meaning to me, I would think of my cadaver's muscles and then imagine my own muscles while waving my arms and legs in front of the bathroom mirror. *Brachioradialis,* I would say to myself as I rotated my forearm and imagined my cadaver doing the same. *Sartorius,* I would think as I sat on a chair and crossed a leg over the opposite knee, imagining this graceful and delicate muscle in my cadaver's thigh and the Roman tailors who gave it its name. The laboratory experience we were struggling with in the afternoons would reinforce, then and forever, the didactic anatomy lectures we heard in the mornings; and to this day, I see my cadaver's body when I envision human anatomy.

We spent two weeks dissecting the arms and legs and began the third week of anatomy with our first exam. During the written portion I spied classmates waving their arms and legs around to jog their memories; they, too, had danced in front of their mirrors. After the written exam we took the practical portion of the test in the laboratories. At various stations our professor displayed dissections from class cadavers with plastic question marks pinned to different structures. The cadavers had been covered so well, except for the vessel or nerve or muscle in question, that it was difficult to figure out what was an arm or a forearm, a leg or a thigh. A timer in the labs went off every two minutes, and as the alarm sounded, each of us scrambled to the next station and struggled to make sense of the disconnected body parts.

In the midst of these cadaveric displays I spied those slender fingers with the coral nail polish and felt a wave of pride. I was pleased with the meticulous work my lab group had done and proud of the beauty of our cadaver's anatomy.

During those early weeks some of my classmates and I began to have dreams about anatomy lab. Some had peaceful dreams in which they held hands with their cadavers or shared a meal. Others were less romantic or downright frightening. My dream, likely fueled by a childhood appreciation of Edgar Allan Poe, remains vivid in my memory. I find myself alone in the laboratory, pacing the hall. The doors of the supply closets that line the hallway swing open suddenly, and cadavers partially dissected and exhibiting signs of putrefaction hang on hooks in each closet. As I try to run away, the closet doors keep opening and closing. Afraid that one of the cadavers will fall on me, I frantically try to escape; but a relentless echoing heartbeat pursues me, growing louder as I run down the hallway.

That morning I woke up exhausted. After a few minutes I realized that the heartbeats I had heard were the reverberations of my own pulse pounding in my ears.

As the weeks passed many of my classmates resorted to black humor. Medical versions of urban legends made the rounds of our laboratories, as they did in medical schools throughout the country. One story was of a medical student who stole a hand and took it to a bar for a variant of the "can you lend me a hand" visual gag. Another story took place at a stadium's urinals with a couple of men, a male medical student, and another stolen anatomic part. One classic legend, probably passed among medical students for generations, had the medical student "friend of a friend" completing dissection on the entire body, only to find upon uncovering the cadaver's face that she had been dissecting her uncle.

Some of my fellow students became increasingly dependent on humor of any kind to lighten the mood in the laboratories and to ease personal anxieties. One group of students brought recordings of old television show theme songs to play while dissecting. Another student adopted the ritual of coming around to each of the four tables in our lab room and playing his air guitar at the beginning of each dissection period. For a while it seemed as if no afternoon could go by without Ben first jamming on that guitar, his thin long face contorted as he lip-synced some classic hard-rock tune playing in his head. Midway through that first semester, however, he and his air guitar suddenly disappeared; Ben had quit medical school.

The daily confrontation with a dead body, the first stranger's body that medical students may have ever examined so closely, marks a point of high anxiety in medical education. Ruth Richardson, in her classic book

Death, Dissection, and the Destitute, writes, "[D]issection requires in its practitioners the effective suspension or suppression of many normal physical and emotional responses to the willful mutilation of the body of another human being." Traditionally medical schools have rarely addressed such psychological concerns; instead educators have only acknowledged the difficulty of mastering the detailed anatomic knowledge. Taking the cues from their teachers, medical students learn to deny their own feelings, depersonalizing the dissection experience and objectifying their cadaver. They strip away the cadaver's humanity, and soon enough they are dissecting not another human being but "the leg" or "the arm."

There are other not-so-subtle clues that reveal the psychological impact of the experience. The frequent cadaver dreams show how profoundly the experience affects the psyche. The use of black humor allows students to deny the significance of any emotional strain. The medical urban legends allow one to hear about someone else's more horrifying experience and thus put one's own experience in a lesser, and therefore more easily palatable, position. At times the denial becomes so great that young medical students are unable to express even their grief. When their emotions are finally released, the manifestations are strangely inappropriate. Ellen Lerner Rothman, M.D., writes in her memoir of her four years at Harvard Medical School:

> At times, it felt as if death were everywhere. In anatomy lab, we finally uncovered the facial shroud and opened the skull to dissect the brain, and that was okay. I talked to a patient who had nearly died the previous evening and would certainly die within the next months, and that was

okay. I came home, and my goldfish had died, and that wasn't okay. I sobbed for half an hour.

Even medical students chosen for their humanitarian qualities and selected from a huge pool of applicants may have their generous impulses profoundly suppressed by their medical education. Some students misinterpret their painful reactions to the dissection process as abnormal and abort their budding medical careers, incorrectly assuming that they have entered the wrong profession.

There are experts in medical education who theorize that the dysfunctional coping mechanisms traditionally used by medical students in their anatomy courses can lead to inappropriately unsympathetic bedside manners. To encourage the development of more effective and desirable attitudes, medical schools have begun to broaden the human anatomy curriculum and have taken steps to mitigate the emotional difficulties. For example, more schools are now holding memorial services for the cadavers at the end of the anatomy course, providing students with an opportunity to express their emotions and gratitude. During these ceremonies, students perform musical pieces and read poems and essays they have written about their cadavers. Some schools have incorporated death-and-dying education into the human anatomy curriculum, drawing on the humanities to generate discussion in small groups and encouraging students to use writing and the fine arts to express their emotions. Still others, plagued by a perpetual shortage of cadavers donated for science, contemplate eliminating dissection altogether, limiting anatomy, and perhaps the student's first encounter with a patient, to a computer-generated experience.

. . .

Over the course of the next week our class dissections centered on the perineal and inguinal, or groin, areas. The layers of muscle and fascia around the rectum, vagina, penis, urethra, and groin overlap and undulate in confusing ways. Despite the careful dissection work on our cadavers, many of us remained frustrated. In fact, it was not until my next-to-last year of surgical residency that I fully understood the many layers and folds of tissue encountered in an inguinal hernia repair.

That fall my classmates and I brought our anatomy texts to the library, the conference rooms, the cafeteria, and the subways and stared at the pictures, trying to commit all the parts to memory. A German anatomy atlas became particularly popular during this segment of our course. Instead of paintings or drawings, this book featured photographs of actual cadaveric dissections. Despite the fact that all the named parts looked ragged from preservation and were of an indistinct beige or gray, some of us believed that these books would help us on exams. On full display wherever we were studying, these atlases would be flipped open to photographs of dissected, spread-eagled, cadaveric male and female genitalia. One classmate realized she had become hardened to these depictions when she looked up from her anatomy books and noticed other passengers on her train commute home moving silently away from her.

Male cadavers were rare that year, so we all crowded around the lab groups who had males to watch the dissection of the male external genitalia. One student read from the *Gray's Anatomy* lab instruction book, the bible of anatomic dissections, while another performed the necessary incisions and maneuvers. It was usually the women who held the scalpel during this part of the dissection. I watched my male classmates wince and shift uncomfortably; there were some areas of the body where we could not, try as we may, separate our own feelings from the science of discovery.

The final maneuver of this section of anatomy would, according to our professor, "bring all the concepts together visually." *Divide the pelvis sagittally,* our *Gray's Anatomy* lab instruction book directed. That afternoon in the laboratories we passed around an electric saw similar to the one my father used for carpentry at home. My lab partners were not sure that we understood what we had read. To our disbelief, we did: we would need to bring the saw down the middle of our cadaver's pelvis and divide it. While this step did indeed expose pelvic anatomy in a way that no other dissection would, I could not bring myself to take the saw to our cadaver. Even after having filleted her arms and legs in previous weeks, I had difficulty with the idea of *sawing* a part of her in two. Realizing that three of us could not do it, Mary, the calm one who would become a family physician, took the saw in hand. She closed her eyes for a moment and then drew the spinning blade down from the center of the symphysis pubis to the strip of flesh between the buttock cheeks. Our cadaver's pelvis, now split, fell apart, the legs turning outward like those of a dancer in the first position. Mary turned off the saw, handed it to the next group of waiting students, and remained silent for the rest of the afternoon.

Since medical school, I have loved gazing at historical lithographs of human anatomy. Tucked away in ancient book stacks in medical libraries, sold in overstocked antiquarian bookstores, or displayed in stands along the Seine in Paris, the pictures are not always anatomically correct, but they are always amusing for their profusion of detail and over-the-top quality. The ones from the Renaissance are often accessorized with ornate calligraphy, the tails of letters curling coyly around the borders. The cadavers are artfully posed, as if about to give a lecture or smell a flower, seemingly unconcerned that their innards are hanging out on full display.

Despite the existence of such lithographs for centuries, public acceptance of human cadaver dissection as a part of medical education is a fairly recent phenomenon. For much of their history, anatomists and physicians worked illegally and surreptitiously, lying, cheating, stealing, and even murdering to further their academic cause. The Council of Tours openly prohibited human dissection in 1163. While their edict was directed more at the practice of dismembering and boiling the remains of dead Crusaders for shipment home, the early Christian beliefs regarding postmortem manipulations were clearly reflected in this decree. After all, the resurrection of the body would be impossible if it had been dissected and therefore desecrated.

During the Renaissance there was a surge of interest in anatomy. Leonardo da Vinci, for example, studied human anatomy in great detail. In 1510 Leonardo completed work that displayed the parallels between human and animal musculature, but his drawings remained unpublished during his lifetime. Andreas Vesalius, the acknowledged father of modern anatomy, performed his own cadaveric dissections and published the seven-volume masterpiece *De Humani Corporis Fabrica* in 1543. His meticulously accurate work revealed that earlier, previously accepted classical authorities such as Galen had been incorrect. Because of religious taboos, the classical anatomists had based their human portraits on animal anatomy.

After the Protestant Reformation in the sixteenth century, London's Royal College of Physicians received the legal authority to dissect human cadavers, but their corpses were limited to those of hanged felons. Dissections at the time were seen as the ultimate punishment for criminals, far worse than a death sentence alone. Even with the corpses of felons, however, the English medical community remained short of cadavers; and surgeons and anatomists resorted to purchasing bodies from grave robbers or "resurrectionists," individuals who exhumed the recently deceased from their graves.

During the nineteenth century Edinburgh was the center of research in anatomy, and Dr. Robert Knox attracted crowds of five hundred or more to his anatomy lectures. The number of aspiring physicians entering the specialty of surgery was also increasing because of the growing respect and honor accorded this profession. The medical school's anatomy and surgery course lasted sixteen months, and students were required to dissect a minimum of three corpses in order to become licensed surgeons. All of these factors further taxed the limited supply of cadavers.

Despite his illustrious reputation, Knox was believed to have remedied this shortage by purchasing bodies from two resurrectionists, William Burke and William Hare. While Burke and Hare did steal corpses from graveyards, they became infamous for having murdered as many as sixteen people in order to sell the bodies. Given the lack of an adequate tissue fixative and ensuing problems of decay, anatomists at the time preferred "fresher" corpses, and the corpses from Burke and Hare were among the most desirable. The two men had devised a technique of asphyxiation that left the cadaver relatively free of any signs of violence. This technique came to be called "burking," a term that eventually worked its way into colloquial English because of the magnitude of the ensuing scandal.

In 1829 Burke was found guilty of murder. His partner, Hare, escaped the death sentence by giving evidence against Burke during the trial. Burke was hanged in front of thirty thousand people, and his body was, rather appropriately, made the subject of a public dissection. His death mask and a wallet made from his tanned skin remain on display at the Anatomy Museum of the Royal College of Surgeons in Edinburgh. As for Dr. Knox, investigators were never able to prove his role in the multiple burkings, but suspicion was so high that the previously esteemed professor was driven out of Edinburgh amid a public frenzy.

In response to the outcry and a subsequent case of burking in 1831, London passed the Warburton Anatomy Act of 1832, which ended the use of dissection as a punishment for murder and gave anatomists unlimited access to unclaimed pauper bodies from workhouses and hospitals. This law ultimately increased the supply of corpses, but many believed that it also transferred the worst punishment for criminals over to the indigent.

In the New World the same social and political forces were at work. While human cadaver dissections took place in America as early as 1638, the demand for cadaver sources began to increase in 1745, when the first formal course in anatomy was offered at the University of Pennsylvania. The only cadavers available legally, however, were the bodies of executed criminals; dissection was used as a form of supra-capital punishment, just as in England. In 1784, for example, to discourage dueling, a Massachusetts law proclaimed that a slain duelist could be either buried without a coffin in a public place and with a stake driven through his body, or given to a surgeon for dissection. Six years later federal judges gained the right to add dissection to the death sentence for murder.

When American medical schools began proliferating in the early nineteenth century, grave robbing became rampant as the demand for cadavers rose. The public became enraged by these acts of desecration and took to the streets in almost a dozen riots between 1765 and 1852. In April 1788, for example, children playing on the streets peered through the windows of the Society of the Hospital of the City of New York and saw medical students dissecting human cadavers. Their parents became outraged when they investigated and saw the dissected corpses. One child's father even discovered that his late wife's corpse, robbed from the grave, was among the dissected. A mob of five thousand stormed the hospital and the jail where several of the doctors had fled to take refuge. A three-day riot ensued, the laboratory was burned down, and seven rioters were killed. The militia finally dispersed the crowd by firing muskets. In response to these riots, New York passed a law in 1789 that allowed doctors to obtain human cadavers without resorting to body snatching.

By the end of the nineteenth century most states had passed laws that allowed medical schools to obtain unclaimed bodies. The impetus for these laws came in 1878, when U.S. Senator John Scott Harrison, the son of President William Henry Harrison and father of President Benjamin Harrison, died and was buried in Ohio. Soon after Senator Harrison's funeral, his son and nephew received word that the body of a family friend, William Devin, had been stolen from its grave and taken to the Medical College of Ohio. The two men went to the anatomy laboratory of the medical school to look for Devin. Instead, they found the body of Senator Harrison about to undergo dissection.

By 1968 all fifty states had adopted the Uniform Anatomical Gift Act. This act ensures that a donor can bequeath his or her body to medical science and education. Since then medical schools have decreased the number of unclaimed bodies used, and the majority of cadavers studied now are the result of conscious and thoughtful decisions made by individuals prior to death. Nonetheless, the ongoing need for bodies and anatomic parts has created latter-day resurrectionists. Two recent cases of body parts being sold—by employees at a California medical school and by a dentist and funeral home director in New York—remind us of nightmares rooted in our collective history.

Despite the difficult history of anatomy, the act of dissecting a human cadaver—of feeling and seeing and holding the human body and its parts—remains fundamental to medical education. For physicians, the experience remains one of the most transformative in their early professional lives.

We moved next in our anatomic journey to the torso. To acclimate our tender hearts to the grisly task, our teachers instructed us to start with the more impersonal back muscles. With fresh blades on our scalpels, we sliced through and peeled away the skin and subcutaneous layers, exposing the pale reddish-brown muscle fibers. The group across from us had a hulking male cadaver who had died in the prime of life. The muscles on his back were large and developed and reminded me of the big chunks of meat I had seen in the butcher's section of the local supermarket. From that point on in my life, I had little enthusiasm for eating red meat; it never tasted the same again.

In contrast, my cadaver had little if any muscular development, and I wondered if my own scrawny back was like hers. Compared to the other cadavers, particularly the males, my cadaver's back muscles seemed barely large enough to have once held her torso erect. Some of her muscular structures were so small that I felt as if I were imagining rather than really seeing the muscles I had read about in my anatomy instruction book. While the larger straps of muscle on my classmates' cadavers were easier to study, I felt possessive of my cadaver and became almost defensive about the tiny strings of tissue that crossed her spine and rib cage.

After dissecting these muscles, we turned our cadavers on their backs and began work on the chest. My three female lab partners and I dissected the breasts particularly gently. We had read about Cooper's ligaments, strings of nearly invisible tissue that suspend the glands, and the complicated ductal system. Much to our dismay, however, we found that the inner tissue of the breast was yellow and globular, not that dissimilar from the fat that we found in other parts of the body. The special ducts and glands that made milk for babies looked just like chicken fat with white, tenuous, connective tissue strings interspersed. It all appeared bland and nondescript.

We peeled away the rest of the skin and subcutaneous tissue to expose the muscles of the chest. The pectoralis major and the pectoralis minor were splayed like magnificent fans across each side. Underneath, the breastbone connected the two halves of the thorax like the hinge on a treasure chest, each rib's tendinous connection like a joint of that hinge. We used another kind of electric saw to perform a median sternotomy, a maneuver that would divide the breastbone along its length, as surgeons do during cardiac operations. Using our index fingers in a technique appropriately referred to as "blunt dissection," we cleared two small spaces just beneath the top and bottom of the sternum; these were the starting and finishing points for our little jigsaw. I revved up the humming motor of the saw, inserted its tip into the divot between our cadaver's collarbones, and drew the vibrating blade along the length of the sternum.

My lab partners and I pulled apart each side of the split breastbone. Underneath we found a pale sac, the pericardium, that enveloped our cadaver's heart. I divided the sac with dissection scissors, thumb and fourth finger in the rings of the instrument. Underneath, a ball of muscle just barely the size of my fist squatted like a bulldog guarding a house. We removed the heart, cutting across its great vessels with large scissors similar to sewing shears, and then spent the rest of the day examining its anatomy. We dissected out the paperlike mitral valve, so named because its two leaflets resemble the pope's miter. Sitting between the left atrium and the left ventricle, the mitral valve is tethered around its periphery by strands of muscle that look like the cords on a parachute. We dissected out the coronary arteries, each barely larger than a sharpened pencil tip. When these arteries are blocked, essential oxygen cannot reach the heart, and this ischemia can result in the death of heart muscle, otherwise known as a myocardial infarction or a heart attack. I stared at these crucial tiny vessels, amazed that people did not suffer heart attacks any earlier in life.

On each side of the now empty pericardium were the lungs, deflated and still. According to our textbooks, each lung was made up of hundreds of millions of microscopic biological balloons called alveoli. Areas that were still inflated were particularly soft, almost velvety. A finger pressed into them left a small glistening depression and made a quiet wet sound, like the one made by a foot on the muddy banks of a pond. Our cadaver's lungs were black and speckled with soot. Initially I thought that the formaldehyde had discolored them, but when I saw the other cadavers' chests—our strapping neighbor's lungs were full and pink—I realized that our cadaver had had a lifetime of cigarettes and some tough city living.

We removed the lungs, cutting across the tubes and vessels that once supplied air and blood. The thoracic cavity, with puddles of formaldehyde settled on the dependent back side, now looked like an emptied, darkened fishbowl. From within we could follow several nerves that extended across the chest wall. The phrenic nerve, whose tiny electrical pulses innervate the muscular diaphragm, seemed hardly like the miserable perpetrator of intractable hiccoughs, but more like a long strand of spaghetti al dente. The imposing aortic arch, that magnificent muscular artery that once carried the oxygenated blood with a great kick from the heart, curved elegantly up toward the brain and then down again toward the abdomen; I could imagine blood jetting from its cavernous hollow into meandering and progressively smaller arteries throughout the body.

We moved downward to the abdomen. We incised the skin, went through the subcutaneous fat, and then dissected out the abdominal wall muscles. Our cadaver's belly was flat, but her abdominal wall hung strangely, given her fine bone structure. There was a looseness to her belly's skin and musculature, as if it had once been round and full, and the muscles here were atrophied and stringy. An old surgical incision traveled in a fine long line from her breastbone to her pubis and distorted the tiny opening in her abdominal wall that would have been her navel.

Once inside her abdominal cavity, we noticed that her intestines seemed oddly tangled. Other cadavers had bowels that were easily manipulated and could slide around freely, as they might have during peristalsis and digestion. My three lab partners and I found ourselves in a maze of bowel loops with no discernible beginning or end. We repeated the mantra of anatomic dissections: *Go from the known to the unknown.* Normally, there is enough consistency in human anatomy that one can recognize newly dissected structures by following the lines of those already identified. We each took a turn trying to make sense of the matted intestines, but the instructions of the anatomy textbook—*Follow the small intestine down to the terminal ileum where you will find the appendix*—confused us even more.

Unlike her orderly arms, back, and chest, our cadaver's abdomen was in disarray. She had no gallbladder. Her omentum, the fatty bib that usually covers the bowels, was gone. Adhesions, scar tissue, distorted her intra-abdominal anatomy, coalescing the delicate individual organs into a big, ugly block.

It was obvious that our cadaver had had surgery of some kind, but what operation could have left her abdominal contents so decimated? My lab partners and I finally went to look at our classmates' cadavers, where the anatomy was more clearly discernible. Each of us was silently disappointed, feeling as if our cadaver had betrayed us and kept the secrets of abdominal anatomy hidden from our probing hands and minds.

By the eighth week of anatomy class, we had dissected our way down to the pelvis. I was immensely curious about the uterus and ovaries. I wanted to see and feel them. What were the organs that held babies and created menstrual periods really like? I remembered my sixth-grade Family Life teacher, Miss Goodwin, explaining menstruation and ovulation. As one of the youngest teachers in my elementary school, Joanna Goodwin had likely been unwillingly corralled into the job of teaching sex education to fifty prepubescent girls. Nonetheless, she managed to be both creative and entertaining. When asked to describe the uterus and ovaries, Miss Goodwin paused momentarily from her fast-paced presentation. Finally, she held both arms up in the air and placed balled-up newspaper in each hand. "Do you see?" she asked us. "My body is the uterus, my arms are the fallopian tubes, and the newspapers are the ovaries."

I half expected to see Miss Goodwin in our cadaver's pelvis, her arms outstretched and her hands grasping two crumpled balls of newspaper. As we delved deeper, my lab partners and I began instead to find balls of hardened tissue. Eager to see the female reproductive organs, we proclaimed the first two balls to be the ovaries. Our cadaver, however, kept bringing forth more balls of tissue, some as small as marbles, others as big as limes. The numerous balls were stuck together, stuck to intestine, stuck to her inner pelvic wall. Some were smooth, but many were like rocks with craggy faces. We called our professor over. He peered into our cadaver's abdominal cavity. "Oh my," he said. "I think she had ovarian cancer."

The ovaries that produced the estrogen that gave our cadaver the feminine features and qualities she cared for so dearly were the very organs that would put an end to her life. At one unknown moment in her life, one of her ovarian cells contorted and mutated and then began to reproduce with unchecked fervor. The anomalous ovarian tissue grew and infiltrated her intestines, causing them to mat together and obstruct. The cancerous tissue produced fluid, ascites, in her belly, which caused the once flat waistline to stretch and bloat and robbed our cadaver of her delicate figure. In death, in that vat of formaldehyde, her ascites had disappeared, so now her stretched abdominal wall hung loosely over her slender frame. The chemotherapy she received in an attempt to hold on to life had left her scalp bare except for a few soft, downy strands. The tumor that had greedily robbed her body of nutrients in its maniacal race to grow had left our cadaver wasted and thin, so that even her back muscles had degenerated into a few measly strings.

Our classmates took a particular interest in the findings in our cadaver's abdomen. As physicians who are meant to cure the ill, we are lifelong students not of the normal but of the abnormal, the anomalies and curiosities of human physiology. Here was a chance to see ovarian cancer in the flesh; for some students it would be their only chance to see the end stages of this disease process. During that long afternoon the anatomy instructors pointed out the irregular agglomerations of tumor in our group's cadaver, and our classmates wandered by and marveled at her intra-abdominal contents. In many ways this scene was a preview of our future as clinicians, when we would, in large groups on clinical rounds, visit living patients. Our preoccupation as medical students with seeing and touching abnormal findings in cadavers already reflected this voyeuristic aspect of our art. Even at the beginning of our schooling, we realized that great clinicians are not just born; they are trained.

By the time my lab partners and I finally uncovered our cadaver's face, we had spent every day for the previous ten weeks in and out of her body. A clear plastic bag encircled her head, and a white muslin cloth, moistened with formaldehyde, clung to the contours that were her eyes, nose, and mouth. I lifted the cloth slowly, starting at the corner that covered her chin. Somehow I felt that seeing her face—her eyes, her lips, and her final expression— would confirm the life I had tried to re-create in my mind. Unlike her abdomen, our cadaver's face was smooth and the skin tight. Her chin appeared exquisitely chiseled, and her lips, still stained with a burnt-orange lipstick, were thin. Despite all the work we had done to the rest of her body over the previous two and a half months, our cadaver looked peaceful, asleep even.

Her eyes were closed. I lifted her right eyelid, wanting to know the color of her eyes, the windows through which she looked out into her world. The eyes, I hoped, would finally tell me the rest of her story. I would be able to look upon her as those who surrounded her during her life had. But there were no eyes under either her right or her left lid, just empty sockets. I had never seen enucleated bare sockets; and instead of being shocked, as I would have imagined, I felt a profound sadness, a kind of void, as if I had been robbed of closure to the imagined life of my cadaver. "She probably donated her corneas after death," said my professor.

Her eyes were not the only things that were taken away before her arrival to us. Her brain, the control center of her soul, had also been removed. "It's being saved for later," said our anatomy professor. "You'll dissect it next semester in neurology lab." The empty cranium, like the hollow eye sockets, looked like a room that had been hastily vacated.

We peeled away the skin on her face, uncovering the nerves and muscles that controlled the expressions she had used over a lifetime. I asked my lab partners to allow me to do this part of the dissection. Holding the small scalpel like a pencil, I separated and lifted the thin facial skin from the underlying muscles, a technique similar to that used in face-lifts. The dissection had to be done meticulously so as not to cut inadvertently any fine facial nerves or vessels. I found the work soothing; over the previous ten weeks I had come to enjoy this technical work of dissection, particularly the finer parts. Moreover, I wanted to spend more time with her face to see if I could piece together other parts of her life.

Unlike many of her other muscles, my cadaver's facial muscles turned out to be beautifully developed. I came to believe that she, even as she approached her death from ovarian cancer, embraced living; the strong muscles of her smile and around her eyes reflected someone who relished life's emotions. While the cancer had eaten away at the rest of her body, these muscles of facial expression survived and even flourished despite the hardships she surely faced.

Unbeknownst to me at that time, my cadaver, my very first patient, was much like my living patients that would follow. Pushed to view their own mortality directly, they too would live the remainder of their own lives that much more fully than the rest of us.

Our final anatomy exam came two weeks later. By this time, dissecting had long since become routine. We spent our free moments at night up in the labs with our cadavers, looking at parts and committing them to memory. If time was short, we ordered pizza after working for a couple of hours, ate quickly in the lab halls, then went back to dissect. The smell of formaldehyde had become a part of life, a badge of pride as we walked by other graduate students who recognized the smell and thus our place as students of medicine. For a brief moment during those twelve weeks we felt like true descendents of our medical forefathers, a part of the history of medicine that has remained unchanged for centuries. We were performing dissections similar to those that had been performed by Vesalius over four centuries before and documenting them within our brains. We came to believe that even in death, the human body contains the secrets of life. And like those great forefathers of medicine, we learned to suppress our instincts of fear and even of repulsion. We pushed those emotions out of our consciousness in order to further medical knowledge.

We had become initiated.

The afternoon after our final exam, I returned to the lab for one last visit with my cadaver. Laboratory technicians had spent the day preparing our cadavers for shipment, but the rooms were now quiet and empty. I opened the familiar latched door underneath the lab bench and pulled out the metal bed.

She was covered neatly in white plastic, ready to move to her final resting place. Through the plastic I touched her forehead, her shoulders, and her hands. I sat in my old jeans and high school T-shirt, thumbing through my memories of her body and the story it told us. I closed my eyes and envisioned her anatomy, referring to it as I would again innumerable times in my future practice. *Thank you,* I thought, feeling at that moment the strong and regular beats at the center of my own chest. *Thank you for your final gift.*

Chapter 2

INTO THE NEXUS

It was nothing like the movies. Sure, someone shouted "Clear!" when the defibrillation paddles were about to go off, and there was a doctor leaning down on the patient's chest and there was another doctor at the foot of the bed calling for medications like lidocaine and epinephrine and atropine. But the coiled EKG reading strips and used syringes strewn about, the lingering smell of burnt flesh where those paddles had emitted their joules, and the naked body that looked not peacefully asleep and perfectly aligned from head to toe but sprawled on the bed as if it had been dropped from the sky—none of this had I ever seen on the screen.

I had just started my third-year clinical coursework. The medical school had sequestered us in lecture halls and laboratories for two years; but now, released into "rotations" or "clerkships," we could roam the hospital wards practically at will and observe and learn from real patients. Our curriculum that year was structured only insofar as we knew we had to rotate a certain number of weeks through six defined specialties. There would be twelve weeks in internal medicine, twelve in surgery, and then six in each of the other major disciplines—obstetrics and gynecology, pediatrics, neurology, and psychiatry. Apart from those rigid requirements, however, the variations were infinite. We could request certain rotations first and others last at up to a half dozen different hospitals. The attending physician groupings within each hospital further complicated our choices. The attendings were the fully trained physicians whose favor we desperately wanted to curry; a well-worded evaluation from the right attending was the key to entering the specialty of our dreams. For my classmates and me, then, positioning ourselves for the best possible specialty-hospital-attending configuration became our obsession of choice.

I was lucky enough to have started with internal medicine at the school's flagship hospital and with a particularly friendly set of attendings. But despite the hours of angst expended on rotation order, hospitals, and attending physicians, my classmates and I would learn that the younger residents were in fact the most important variable. Most of our days and nights would be spent trailing these trainees; some were first-rate teachers, others world-class slave drivers. And in the end, none of these doctors was more influential that year than the interns, those first-year residents who, in the rigid academic medical hierarchy, stood only slightly higher than we did.

I spent the earliest weeks of that summer glued to
Manny, a gangly intern from New York. Manny loved clinical medicine. He thrived on the minutiae of the work,
inebriated by his mastery of this professional Trivial Pur-
suit. He delighted in the way the multisyllabic names of
esoteric diseases rolled off his tongue. He quoted from the
latest medical journal reports and reeled off dozens of laboratory values for each of his patients, like a boy spouting
the statistics of his favorite baseball team. What Manny
loved most, however, was the Socratic method of teaching.
Despite having graduated only a month earlier from medical school himself, Manny could quickly assume the air of
a distinguished visiting professor. And as he pontificated,
my mind wandered; I often found myself staring at his
cherry-sized Adam's apple, hypnotized by its rhythmic
bobbing over the ridges of his trachea.

Inevitably, at some point during his discourse Manny
would pause, a sign that he was about to ask me a question. My mind had become more sievelike since starting
medical school; I barely retained any old information and
almost certainly would not be able to summon forth the
scattered bits I had achingly memorized the night before.
Manny's pregnant pauses would cause me to start, and I
would frantically try to retrieve my thoughts from their
hypnotic attachment to his neck. By the time Manny
finally posed the question, a torrent of incorrect answers
would spew forth from my mouth. Manny was delighted by
my incompetence; each wrong answer was another opportunity for him to teach. In my mind, however, these ses-
sions became the unnerving private confirmation of my two
worst fears. First, my ineptitude would prevent me from
ever graduating from medical school. And second, I was
only one memory flaw away from inadvertently killing a
patient, even if with the best of intentions.

Nonetheless, I enjoyed hanging around Manny. I liked that he was from the East Coast, like me, and thought that everyone around him talked funny. I liked that he really seemed to enjoy caring for his patients, even the ones who had odd smells emanating from their person and who hated having to talk to an intern and medical student instead of to the attending physician. And I liked that he found having a medical student tagging along at all hours of the day and night more amusing than annoying.

The very first time he turned professor with me, Manny taught me about the different classes of drugs used to treat hypertension. Abruptly, in the middle of his lecture, he stopped speaking and began grinning. "What's up, Manny?" I asked, half afraid that I had missed something by spacing out on his Adam's apple.

"Do you know, Pauline, that someday you'll be sitting here in my chair and teaching some medical student?" He paused and smiled, tickled by the thought. "And maybe you'll be teaching them exactly what I'm teaching you." His smile became enormous.

During our nights on call together, Manny usually sent me to sleep after midnight so that he could dispense with the final details of his work alone. One night fairly early on in that summer, however, Manny knocked on the call room door about a half hour after he had sent me to sleep. "Hey, Pauline! There's a code!" The heart of a patient somewhere in the hospital had stopped, and a team of doctors and nurses was trying to resuscitate the patient. Manny's eyes were sparkling, and he kept swinging the call room door back and forth in a kind of nervous fidget. The light from the hallway flashed into the room every time he opened the door, only to disappear a moment later when he closed it. I tumbled out of bed, as much to stop Manny's makeshift strobe light as to see the code. "This will be a good learning experience for both of us," he said as I pulled on my short white medical student coat.

Outside the call room I heard the hospital operator on the PA system, her voice reverberating through the deserted corridors. "Code Blue, Room 842, Jackson Pavilion. Code Blue, Room 842, Jackson Pavilion," she announced over and over again in a strained whisper, as if she knew it was the middle of the night but had no idea that her voice was echoing over hospital loudspeakers. Manny and I ran up the back stairs to the eighth floor, where lights were flashing in the hall. A crowd of residents, nurses, respiratory therapists, and nursing aides spilled forth from the door to Room 842, and more hospital staff, like us, kept emerging from the elevators and stairwells, wide-eyed, panting, and running toward the room.

A trio of nurses pushed an unwieldy metal cart through the hallway and straight into the crowd of people. "Out of our way!" one of the nurses shouted. "We've got the code cart!" The group at the doorway parted just long enough for the cart and three nurses to get through and then reconverged, blocking access once again. Once inside the room the nurses broke the flimsy plastic locks that secured the drawers and the defibrillator paddles and began drawing up dozens of medications into syringes.

Standing near the door, I recognized a couple of other medical students in the room who had also come for the "learning experience." We smiled and shrugged our shoulders to one another; we had no idea what was about to take place but figured it was worth being up. One of the nurses at the code cart eyed the crowd like a tiger about to jump its prey. "All nonessential people, get out of the room!" she growled. The crowd backed off. I tried to move in for a better view, but the nurse, as if she had caught me, then roared, "Medical students and other folks who are not helping here, please get out of the room!" I slinked back to the rear of the crowd.

It was two o'clock in the morning. The residents and interns, who had taken off their street clothes and now wore hospital scrubs, seemed to have aged a decade since I last saw them twelve hours earlier. Smeared mascara on the women and an evening's worth of dark growth on the men accentuated their fatigue. Only the lone blond ponytail of the resident in charge of the code bounced effortlessly at this hour.

I had seen this senior resident, Karen, during the day at one of the medical conferences. She was one of the best residents in her class, and now, with only a year left of training she carried herself with the confidence of someone on the verge of becoming an attending physician. I was always in awe of her poise and the way she presented her patients' cases; she knew exactly what to do and how things would turn out. My medical school friends who were part of her team worshipped her, and we were amazed that only a little over three years ago she had been a medical student like us at this school.

On my tiptoes and from outside the room's door, I watched Karen standing alone at the foot of the bed and calling out orders. Her night on call had probably been busy; she was still wearing her black-and-white-houndstooth dress. Her ponytail bobbed as she looked from the cardiac monitor to the patient, then to the other residents and nurses. Even from beyond the doorway, I could see her hands shaking. In fact, her whole body shivered.

I did not recognize the patient on the bed, but I could tell he was male; the resuscitation team had pulled off his hospital gown and all remaining shreds of clothing. He had a few gray hairs and the gnarled joints of an arthritic patient. The oddest part of him, however, was his skin color. It was blue, making it difficult for me to figure out his ethnicity. Even from a distance, I knew that with that bluish tinge, his skin probably felt a whole lot cooler than mine.

The bed was tilted head down in Trendelenburg position to encourage blood from the feet and legs to move toward the man's brain. The resuscitation team had rolled his body onto a hard board that provided counterresistance to the CPR thrusts against his chest. But on top of the soft hospital bed, every push down on his chest caused his torso to move ever more slightly askew on the board, until a final thrust pushed the man's body completely off the board. Each time, the team heaved his body back on, struggling against the softness of the underlying mattress and the downward pull of the Trendelenburg position; but even after they had successfully done so, an arm would swing out, or a leg would hang over, or the whole body would just go sliding down toward the head of the bed. After a few rounds of this the team gave up, trying instead just to get as much of his torso on the board as possible and leaving the extremities to their own devices, dangling in four different directions.

As I watched two residents poke needles into the patient's groin in vain attempts to get blood, I felt relieved to be a mere medical student with no responsibility and no skills to add. On the fifth poke, the residents hit a vessel and pulled back what they believed was blood from the femoral artery. The fluid in their syringe was almost black. They showed it to Karen before one of the nursing aides grabbed it to take to the laboratory. Karen shivered again and then looked at the electronic green line of the cardiac monitor. The pattern on the screen kept jumping erratically up and down, like a hapless dancer on a futile search for the music's beat.

Karen closed her eyes. I imagined that she was visualizing the decision tree for cardiac resuscitations, translating the steps into orders for the rest of the team. I thought about my own review of advanced cardiac life support earlier that month; it had been the first assignment of the clerkship.

Ventricular tachycardia, a rhythm with an EKG tracing like the teeth of a saw, needs the drug amiodarone and then a shock from the defibrillator. Ventricular fibrillation, an even worse rhythm that is barely like a squiggle, needs intravenous epinephrine and 200 joules from the defibrillator pads. Increase to 300 joules if there is no response in the heart's rhythm, and further increase to 360 joules if no regular rhythm returns, but increase no farther. Check the levels of acid in the blood and give shots of intravenous calcium, magnesium, and maybe even some bicarbonate, but not too much because that could worsen the patient's status. Make sure no one is touching the patient when the paddles go off—shout "Clear!"—otherwise someone else's heart might be shocked into a life-threatening rhythm. And don't forget to always have someone pushing on the chest, doing CPR, between shocks.

Finally, Karen turned to the crowd. Her face was colorless. "Does anyone have any more ideas here?" she asked. The three nurses at the code cart looked at one another and shook their heads. The respiratory therapist at the head of the bed silently shifted his weight from one foot to the other as he continued squeezing the bag that pushed oxygen into the patient's lungs. Manny, who had gone in to help by pumping on the patient's chest, stopped to wipe his brow. When he lifted his arm to his forehead, I saw the large round sweat stain at his armpit.

Karen smiled weakly in response to everyone's silence. Hers was not the smile of joy but the kind forced against tears.

Ten minutes later the attending physician blew into Room 842. "I'm the attending!" he shouted. "Let me in here! Let me in here!" There were lines across his cheeks; he had gone directly from his bed, to his car, then to the hospital. Everyone stepped back, and even Manny stopped pumping on the patient's chest to look up. "Keep doing CPR!" the attending barked at Manny.

Karen walked over to the attending physician and relayed the events leading up to the code. His bluster slowly dissipated; whatever his therapeutic interventions had been for this patient, they had obviously failed.

"Do you want to call the code now?" Karen asked. The patient's monitored heart rhythms had long since degenerated into limp squiggles, more the consequence of drugs and joules than of any remaining life force.

"We have to keep going in case there's a chance," the attending snapped back. I watched him pace around the room, shout orders to the resuscitation team, and quietly curse at himself, at Karen, and even at the patient for the now inevitable outcome. After thirty minutes, he looked at the nurse who had been recording the code. "Let's call it," he said and then walked away.

The floor and bed were littered with EKG tracings, empty medication vials, and stray needles and syringes. Blood stained the sheets of the patient's bed. There were oval burn marks on his chest from the defibrillator paddles. A few nurses and aides lingered behind to clean the patient's body and room. Another nurse called out for the ward secretary, asking her to telephone the patient's family so that the attending physician could inform them of the news.

The crowd dispersed quickly. Many immediately began to discuss the next set of medical tasks: admitting the new patient who was waiting in the emergency room, checking the results of midnight radiology studies, writing a few more orders.

As I walked back to the call room with Manny, both of us silent, all I could think of was that this code was nothing like the movies. It was messy, it was chaotic, and in the end, someone had really died.

Even as a child, I knew that doctors had different sensibilities. One of my uncles is a urologist, and while he has the same complexion, male pattern balding, and squared-off fingers as my father, the similarities stop there. My father, for example, crammed his home office with bills and crates of computer cards, but my uncle littered his with medical journals that displayed diseased human organs and disconnected parts. The childhood scrapes that sent my parents running to phone our pediatrician elicited, at most, a gruff snort from my uncle.

When I was in junior high school, I used to ask my uncle on his biannual visits what the worst thing he had seen was. Like most adolescents I had a tentative fascination with all things gross. A part of me wanted to see if I could stand my uncle's stories; even more, I wanted to see how much it would take to disgust my uncle. But there was never the slightest hint of revulsion from him. Instead, on the living room sofa, with my younger brother toddling about in front of us, he would begin recounting the stories of patient afflictions. His glasses would slide down his nose; and each time I gasped, he would look over at me, surprised, that flat clinical voice never for a moment wavering.

Sociologists, anthropologists, and medical educators themselves have long known that medical students must learn to endure and even embrace what might be considered by others to be difficult or even ghastly. They must reconcile incompatible ideals or "counterattitudes"—values as diametrically opposed as detachment and concern, certainty and uncertainty, and humanism and technology. Like adolescents searching for a sense of identity, medical students will vacillate between each extreme. They may be overly concerned at one moment but then become coolly detached in the next.

Ultimately they will settle at a comfortable equilibrium point, and this act of creating a new moral paradigm—detached concern, secure uncertainty, and humanistic technology—marks an important step in the transformation of the lay medical student into full-fledged professional physician.

Medical students start the process of professionalization as anyone thrown into daily contact with the sickest people in a community might: with a sense of shared dread. As a medical student on the wards, I felt awkward enough because of my negligible clinical experience, but it was that shared vulnerability with patients that made me feel completely incompetent. The older nurses administered vaccinations in a second as I winced in unrestrained empathy; when it was my turn to give the shots, I moved so slowly and shook so much that I only worsened the patients' pain. When holding a scalpel for the first time in the operating room, I could not bear to press the sharp blade against another living person's flesh and so left a negligible scratch on the patient's belly; at that rate it would have taken all day to complete the skin incision. During my pediatrics rotation I contracted every viral illness from the children on the wards; the more experienced residents, wary of the effects of my uncontrollable hacking on fearful parents, handed me a mask every time we entered a hospital room. I felt more like another pediatric patient than a competent and immune doctor.

In those earliest days on the ward, any little

accomplishment—the first successful intravenous catheter placement, the first written prescription, the first independent patient workup—helped boost my budding professional self-image. Still, what I wanted most desperately was to *become* a doctor; I wanted to learn not just clinical work but clinical sensibilities.

I found myself hungering for more procedures—blood draws, stitches, tube insertions—anything where practice would not only make perfect but would also numb my instinctive responses. I was first fascinated with patients whose predicaments were as far from my own as statistically possible—those afflicted with oddball one-in-a-million diseases—but then I pushed myself to become more interested in the one-in-500,000, then one-in-250,000, then one-in-100,000 cases. To prove that I was as capable of resisting normal fatigue as the next doctor, I forced myself to imitate my interns' hours, staying up for forty-eight hours, sleeping for six, then appearing more enthusiastic than ever the next morning on rounds.

But dying patients were a different matter. It seemed that to those above me—the fourth-year students, the interns, the residents, and the attending physicians—dying patients were clinical events. I tried desperately to be like the older residents—"Great! Another code! Another opportunity to learn!"—but seeing patients die bothered me.

I probably never would have admitted it to anyone back then, but I did not believe that death was merely clinical. In my mind dying had as much to do with fate as with biology. I had even thought about my own death in those terms.

Try as I might, I could not act like my residents. That great passing of life was too sacred; it was nearly magical. Death was an immutable moment in time, locked up as much in our particular destiny as in the time and date of our birth.

My mother and father arrived in the United States some three years before my birth. Part of a cadre of young Taiwanese scholars who graduated from the country's most competitive university, they had secured graduate student scholarships at prestigious American universities and then passed the grueling Taiwanese national exam for exit visas. In old family albums there are photos of my parents at the airport in Taipei as they are about to start their lives abroad; each is adorned with leis of white orchids and flanked by dozens of relatives squinting against the tropical sun.

Within three years, however, my parents' lives were as bleak as the January skies of New England. They lived in the third-floor apartment of a poorly maintained Cambridge triple-decker, were regular clients of the local Salvation Army thrift store, and ate lunches of a homemade steamed bread that my mother made yellow and marginally more nutritious by adding an egg. My father worked as a teaching assistant, while my mother waited tables and then, as a bank clerk, handled the money that others seemed to have so much of and she so little. And each month they dutifully sent most of their income to my father's struggling family.

In those early years together, their single greatest investment was a used bike. Even during the snowy winters, to save on the ten-cent bus fares, they rode to school together on that bike. My father pedaled up front, and my mother, head covered in a scarf and arms wrapped around my father's waist, sat sidesaddle on the back fender.

It was into this graduate student poverty on a cool fall

morning in 1964 that I was born, with as much parental dread as loving anticipation. It did not help matters that I was also born backward: feet first. The youngest and most inexperienced doctor at the hospital attended my mother initially, but the parade of obstetricians became more professorial as it became clearer I was unlikely to turn around in utero before emerging. My mother, who did not know enough English to understand their concerned pronouncements, clung to a piece of moist gauze, quietly clenching it between her teeth as I descended. She had delivered, my grandmother later commented, like a Japanese princess.

Despite their limited incomes, one of the first things my parents did after my birth was to send a small bundle abroad. I have often suspected that this act was a splurge, but to my parents mailing this package was more important than any winter bus ride, cafeteria-bought meal, or brand-new coat. To them, it was as significant as my birth.

When my maternal grandmother received this package in Taipei, she brought the contents—a letter with the date and exact time of my birth and a piece of clothing that my mother had worn during her pregnancy—to an elderly man who lived at the edge of the city. I have often imagined him: a wizened individual in black cotton shoes with wispy strands of white hair growing from his chin, a curling pinkie fingernail, and a sleepy expression accentuated by the drag of gravity. According to my parents that old man, a fortune-teller famous in Taiwan, inspected the items and then began writing on a small scroll in meticulous Chinese script about the trials and tribulations of my life to come. He commented on my health, chronicled my studies, and described the riches that would and would not come my way. He wrote that I would be a "wild horse," and because the "traveling star" had ascended during my birth, I would have difficulty staying put.

At the end of the scroll, the old man wrote a few characters alluding to my death. There are, however, no specifics: no date, no time, and not even a word about the way in which I will die.

I have never seen the scroll. Somewhere along its journey from Taipei to that Cambridge triple-decker and to the half dozen other places my parents eventually moved, it was lost. Nonetheless, those predictions have become woven into my life like a birthmark—always present but obvious only when I care to look.

In the course of my life, I have tended to look to that scroll pretty frequently—when I went to college, when I went to medical school, and when I moved around for my clinical training. I thought about those predictions when I got married, and they were foremost on my mind in the birthing room when I first heard the times of my twin daughters' births.

But the scroll and the fortune-teller came back to me most vividly one night during my third year of medical school. It was the night I first pronounced a patient dead.

I was spending the month working with Bill, a shy, doughy intern with a reputation for clinical efficiency and a weakness for food. Each morning Bill, the members of the medical team, and I left rounds with prodigious amounts of "scut"—Some Clinically Useful Tasks—to do. From the moment we dispersed, Bill was a man on a mission, checking off each item on his personal scut list— draw blood, write orders, schedule studies, retrieve reports—with unerring efficiency. By two o'clock every afternoon, and several hours before everyone else on the team, Bill would be done with his scut. Without fail, I could find him celebrating on a call room bed, surrounded by his beeper, portable television, and a few bags of junk food.

One night when we took call together, Bill and I sat to eat the last pieces of room-temperature pizza that Joe, another intern, had ordered. Joe was the anti-Bill intern: inefficient, emaciated, and often harsh. And his pizza slices looked like triangles of midwestern prairie—flat and beige—bordered by a crust burnt to a flaky black. Bill bit into a slice and then spit it into the trash. "Never ask anyone like Joe to order your food," he said, gagging on the aftertaste. "If you want the best food, you need to ask your patient with high blood pressure, heart disease, and diabetes where they would go if they wanted to cheat." He patted his soft belly and smiled. "Or you can ask someone like me."

From that night on, and under Bill's tutelage, I took charge of ordering dinner for the on-call team. After a few of my dinners, some of the residents tried to get me to take call with them by assigning me the clinical responsibilities I craved—a new patient to work up, a blood draw to perform, another set of lost X-ray films to hunt down. Others pulled me aside during call for impromptu mini-lectures on the patient diseases we were seeing on the wards. While I knew that these were self-interested forms of appreciation, I couldn't have cared less. Nothing made my medical student heart sing more than hearing a resident ask, "Hey, where's Pauline?" even if it was only for dinner.

Best of all, by the end of that month, I had become a miniature Bill, the medical student prototype of clinical efficiency, and my greatest triumph occurred on the next-to-last day that I worked with Bill. Completed scut list in hand, I spent the hour before evening rounds curled up in the chair next to Bill's call room bed, licking the potato chip salt off my fingers and celebrating the deviousness of his favorite soap opera diva.

. . .

Sometime in the middle of that month, during another call night together, Bill paged me to the ICU. "Hey, Pauline," Bill said when I arrived. "One of the patients just died. The nurses need a death note, so they can send the body down to the morgue and get the room cleaned."

Bill signaled for me to follow him. I remembered my grandfather and my gross anatomy cadaver; and my grandfather was so beloved and my cadaver submerged in formaldehyde for so long that neither could count as a *real* dead body. I thought about the man who had died during the resuscitation and wondered if this patient would be blue, too. As we walked toward the room, I remembered a story from junior high school: a fellow hospital volunteer was transporting a patient's dead body to the autopsy labs when the corpse suddenly sat up on the gurney, causing the candy striper to scream and run away. "It was rigor mortis," a doctor later told me. Now I wanted to know how long it would be before rigor mortis set into this body.

But when I looked over at Bill to ask, he seemed bored, tired, and not the least bit interested in medical student stupid questions in the middle of the night. And no one else around us seemed to care, either. A few residents straggled by. Bill looked at them, raised the dead patient's chart in the air in greeting, and said simply, "Death note." In reply, they rolled their eyes and kept walking. The nurses at the station continued to write their progress notes and dispense medications. The unit secretary announced she was going on break and asked a nurse to cover the phone while she was away.

Bill and I walked into the patient's room together. I could hear the soft buzz of the fluorescent lights overhead and the echo of our footsteps. The patient was an elderly

Caucasian man who had small islands of white flakes on his gray skin. His parched lips had relaxed to form the letter O, and his tongue was lolling to one side.

Bill pointed to the mouth. "Q sign," he whispered, opening his own mouth and letting his tongue hang out on one side. I spied a few beads of sweat just above Bill's eyebrows. "Go to the last page on the chart," he said, wiping the sweat away with the back of his hand.

"Okay," I whispered back, not quite sure why both of us were whispering.

"There are three things you need to check when you declare death," Bill said. His efficiency was creeping in; he had a way of reducing every clinical task to a series of steps. "First, there have to be no spontaneous heartbeats." Bill placed the bell of his stethoscope against the center of the patient's chest, listened for a minute, and then motioned for me to do the same.

I heard the whooshing of my own pulse, the "ocean" in an empty seashell.

After a few seconds Bill continued his whispered instructions. "Then you need to make sure there are no spontaneous breaths." I wondered how long the two of us would have to stand in that room watching the dead man's chest, waiting for it to rise and fall. Before I could ask, however, Bill snapped the stethoscope earpieces back in his ears and placed the bell once more against the man's chest. I copied him obediently and again heard only the ocean.

Satisfied by the silence, Bill shoved his stethoscope back into his coat pocket. "Lastly," he said, his whisper slowly giving way to a normal talking voice, "there must be no response to painful stimuli."

"What do you mean by 'painful stimuli'?" I wanted to ask, but before I even opened my mouth, Bill was twisting the papery skin of the dead man's hand between his own fleshy thumb and index finger. "You can pinch their skin, you can roll a pencil against their fingernails, you can pinch their nipples. Anything that gets a rise out of people." He released the skin and looked at me; it was my turn to inflict pain. I reached for the part of the man closest to me and least intrusive: his right middle finger. I squeezed the nail bed.

Bill began laughing. "That wouldn't get a rise out of me, and I'm a lot more alive than this guy." Bill grabbed my hand and laid it over the dead man's left nipple. I couldn't bear to squeeze that small pointed piece of flesh, so I tweaked some of the skin just to the side. It was warm, pliant even, but felt unconnected, like the skin of supermarket chicken.

Bill pointed to the patient's chart. "Write this," he directed. "It's what you need to write in death notes, just a few sentences. 'No spontaneous heartbeat. No spontaneous breaths. No response to painful stimuli. Patient pronounced dead at . . .' " Bill stopped and looked up at the clock.

It was 2:23 a.m. The scraggly fortune-teller popped into my head. I saw him dipping his pointed brush into the inkwell and pulling small, measured strokes across the paper.

"What do you think?" Bill asked me. "He's probably been dead for about fifteen minutes." He paused for a moment. "Why don't you write that the patient died at 2:08 a.m.?"

The old fortune-teller disappeared.

Dutifully, I wrote what Bill said and then signed my name. Bill countersigned the note and walked back with me to the nursing station. "See, Pauline," he said as he put away the chart, "now you know how to declare someone dead." He smiled broadly. "Isn't it easy?"

I nodded.

That night I could not fall asleep. For the first time since beginning medical school, I felt like a real doctor. I heard over and over again in my head: "Dr. Chen pronounced the patient dead at 2:08 a.m.," and I kept thinking about the ten minutes I had spent in the room with Bill. I wanted to relive every detail of what I had done.

By the morning I was exhausted. I went on rounds, did my scut, but in my sleep-deprived haze began to feel off-kilter. The more I thought about the previous night, the less I felt doctorly. I began to feel angry with Bill for reducing a man's death to three steps and guilty for being complicit in the act. I wanted to go back to the chart, tear out my note, and write something more appropriate, longer, and more thoughtful than three steps. The more I thought about that death note, the more discombobulated I became—it was as if my world, spinning around along its usual trajectory, had slowed to a wobble.

That afternoon, as I was about to find Bill, the old man popped into my head again, as he would in the future every time I looked at a clock to pronounce a patient dead.

And suddenly, I understood why. I had insinuated my hand into that mysterious nexus of stars and fate and destiny, and I had reduced that great passing of life into an arbitrarily calculated moment in time.

Chapter 3

SEE ONE, DO ONE

Every morning around 7:20 in the hospital where I trained, the junior residents would gather in the cafeteria for breakfast. Work rounds would be done, and the senior residents and chiefs would have already gone off to the operating rooms for the day, leaving us junior residents with lists of scut to complete before evening rounds.

In the midst of overwhelming days, these fifteen minutes in the cafeteria were a symbol of our united defiance. We would put all but the most urgent pages on hold and stake out the same section of tables on the far end of the cafeteria. Together, we would cavalierly devour what we called the "cardiac special," an intoxicating, heart-stopping, artery-clogging glob of eggs, cheese, and sausage between a grilled kaiser roll—the caloric equivalent of a day's worth of meals—and then poke fun at those attendings and senior residents in whose thrall we normally cowered. We learned to squeeze a day's worth of socializing and gossip into fifteen minutes, and by the end of those brief breakfasts, we would trudge back to the wards, our bellies and souls filled.

Inevitably these hurried conversations ended up centering on work—how much there was, what we had to do, and how our lives were unbelievably difficult because of it. We would take turns spinning our own tales of woe; it was, after all, a personal badge of honor not only to have lived through such horrors but also to have survived intact enough to join everyone else at the breakfast table. There were stories about "crashing" patients, those whose clinical courses took a sudden turn for the worse, traumas that involved half a dozen victims, and, of course, chief residents or attending surgeons who reprimanded unreasonably. All of us would talk, each with a horror story worse than the others, the subtext always being that the person who told the worst tale was the hardest-working, and therefore best, intern.

One morning late in my internship, the intern taking care of Mr. Roberts began talking. We were all quiet because we knew that no one could outdo him. John Roberts had been in the hospital longer than we had been interns, and every one of us dreaded the month when we would have to take care of him. Mr. Roberts had a particularly intractable case of Crohn's disease, an inflammatory disease of the bowel that can result in pain, diarrhea, bleeding, and blockage of the intestines. Mr. Roberts had had several blockages and operations previously, but on this hospital admission, his blocked bowel was so inflamed that even the gentlest surgeon's fingers wreaked chaos in their path.

He never healed. One loop of his bowel stuck up against the wall of his abdomen and developed a fistula, a tunnel between that bowel and the outside that leaked abdominal contents through the nearest opening, his incision wound. Copious amounts of fluid with ribbons of green bile and flecks of sloughed tissue splashed daily onto Mr. Roberts, breaking up any tenuous skin cells that tried to cover both the wound and the fistula. In an effort to decrease the amount of fluid coming out from his bowel, the medical staff forbade Mr. Roberts from eating and nourished him instead with bags of intravenous nutrition. The nurses set up suction tubing to clear the liters of secretion, but his dressings still saturated quickly, turning the skin around the wound into a waterlogged mess. Mr. Roberts thus passed the days alone in his hospital room hooked up, sucked on, and bathing in his own intestinal contents.

By the time my turn came to care for him, Mr. Roberts had been hospitalized for six months. I dreaded going into that room. Every morning when I went in to examine him, he looked neither at me nor at what I was doing. The shades were always drawn, and the smell of skin soaked in small bowel contents, a strangely sweet, less intense version of rotting pears, permeated the room. His answers to my awkward attempts at conversation were usually terse. And I always felt like part of the cause of his misery. Even if I had not been at the operation and even if there had been no other alternative than surgery, entering that room made me feel more a part of the brethren of medicine than any other thing I did that year.

He was thin, that much was easy to tell from the gaunt figure that lay on the bed. He had a pleasant face—oval but chiseled by male hormones. And he was tall; his legs were always bent up, and even then his feet hit the end of his bed. The nurses had miraculously rigged up a way to move all his accoutrements, but I saw him outside the room only once, escorted by a nurse who pushed along the pole and cart that carried the bags of intravenous nutrition and the tangle of suction tubing. I was shocked but recovered quickly enough to stop and say hello. Mr. Roberts looked at me for a moment, as if he was trying to focus his eyes on my face and could not quite remember who I was. He smiled and then, looking at my white coat, said, "Hi, Doctor."

So when the intern who was in charge of Mr. Roberts that month began to talk, none of us dared utter a word. Instead we sat mute, eating our breakfasts and relieved for once not to be the best intern.

Mr. Roberts was not getting better, and the surgeon in charge was contemplating surgery. It was a drastic step; Mr. Roberts would have to gamble on the slim hope that surgery would help, even though the odds were that it would only complicate things further. Or he could choose to live out the rest of his life in his current state. Even at our tender ages, the choice seemed excruciatingly difficult for a man who was not yet fifty. As the intern continued to speak, his beeper went off. He looked at it. "It's Roberts's floor. I bet it's his nurse." We watched our fellow intern as he took one last bite from his roll and started walking out of the cafeteria, coffee cup in hand.

John Roberts died a week later without the surgery. His death was the topic of discussion the next morning at breakfast, and a few of the second-year residents weighed in with their opinions. "You know every class of interns has a patient like Roberts, someone who is in the hospital for the entire year," said one of them. "We had a guy like that, too." The two other second-year residents nodded, smiling and remembering their "John Roberts." By virtue of the several thousands of hours of clinical experience they had acquired in the year before us, they seemed infinitely wiser than we interns were.

Another second-year resident began to talk. "The key," he said, "is not being the poor sucker that's on the service when the guy dies. You do everything to keep that guy alive until you rotate off-service."

The interns all looked at him. We leaned in, waiting for the punch line.

The resident took a bite of his breakfast sandwich and began waving it around, like a professor at his chalkboard. "You do everything to keep the guy alive because you don't want to be the poor bastard who has to go through a year of medical charts to dictate the death note."

We all sat back. All of us had bumbled through discharge dictations on patients we hardly knew; it required wading through the charts late at night after all the ward work had been done and piecing together events from scrawled, usually illegible notations. For John Roberts's dictation, I envisioned our fellow intern sitting in front of a colossal tower of charts for an entire sacred weekend off.

The following year when I heard that the next intern class's "John Roberts" had died, I remembered my Mr. Roberts and the awkward morning visits, the smell of his bowel contents on skin, and the gnawing discomfort I felt every time I left his room to eat the breakfast he never could. Two years later, when another similar patient died, my best friend in residency, Celia, and I spent a few minutes over dinner remembering Mr. Roberts and discussing his medical case before we went off to see our next patient.

Over the years, however, as more patients passed through my life, I found that my memories of John Roberts became less sharp, that he became less unique to me, less sad, and even less frightening. Mr. Roberts—his leaking fistula, the darkened room, and his seemingly endless hospital stay terminated only by death—nearly disappeared from my recall banks. Instead, after a few years I recalled only one thing: the breakfast the morning after. Whenever a patient like John Roberts died in the hospital, the first words out of my mouth were "Consider yourself lucky that you aren't the poor bastard to do the death dictation."

I never intended to make my living among the dying. When I entered medical school, I dreamed of helping people. And for me, *helping* meant *saving* lives. I imagined a clinic filled with grateful, cured, modern-day Lazarus equivalents. I also convinced myself that my undergraduate background in medical anthropology would make me more empathic than other physicians; my patients would not only be physically cured but would be emotionally healed in culturally relevant ways.

As it turns out, my dreams about my future medical career were not that different from those of most medical students. Premedical students overwhelmingly believe that as physicians they will be able to cure and help their patients. Few choose this career to care for the dying; instead, they believe they will save others from the inevitability of death.

Sherwin Nuland postulates in his book *How We Die* that "of all the professions, medicine is one of the most likely to attract people with high personal anxieties about dying. We became doctors because our ability to cure gives us power over the death of which we are so afraid." Attracted to medicine in part because of our own particular anxieties, we may be a self-selected lot who eagerly suppress these fears as we adopt a professional ethos that embraces denial.

Once we are accepted into medical school, we advance through the ranks, becoming medical students, then interns, then residents, and then perhaps subspecialty fellows. In this modern apprenticeship we take our cues from the fully trained attending physicians who serve as our clinical professors, mimicking their thought processes, preferences, and even attitudes. The attendings take their teaching responsibilities and the professional hierarchy quite seriously. Charles Bosk, a medical sociologist, writes that "[the] power of attendings in the system of everyday controls is truly remarkable." In some specialties that hierarchy is so powerful that any perceived deviations from attending physicians, in action or even words alone, can become grounds for job termination.

As young students and doctors in the midst of profound sleep deprivation and chaotic personal lives centered on work, we are eager to find easy truths or at least comfortable lessons in patient care. Soon enough, however, we discover that death among patients is an inevitable part of our profession. We look to our attending physicians for guidance and we learn that many of them have not only their own difficulties in dealing with death but also little insight into how these attitudes affect the care they give terminal patients. Even our textbooks, usually overflowing with data, provide us with little or no help with the dying.

Thus, without guidance or advice, few of us ever adequately learn how to care for patients at the end of life. We end up sifting through our own experiences with precious little support, and we watch patients die, sometimes directly under our watch and always despite all of our best efforts and all that we have learned. For many of us, it is a rite of passage that is painful and terrifyingly lonely; years afterward, even decades afterward, we cannot forget our first patients.

I was in my final year of medical school and was spending a month in the medical intensive care unit learning about critical care when Juliette, an elderly woman with pneumonia, arrived. Juliette's infection had taken over most of her normal lung tissue; from the moment we admitted her into the ICU, she required a mechanical ventilator to breathe and thus remained fully sedated.

To those of us on rounds that first morning, Juliette looked like the classic "LOL," or little old lady—white-haired and with finely crinkled paper-thin skin. Her eyes were closed, and it would have been hard for passersby to distinguish her from the dead except for the regular beeps coming from her cardiac monitor. Because Juliette's medical condition was a "bread and butter" type of case—elderly people with pneumonia were admitted again and again during the Chicago winters—the resident in charge of the ICU assigned me to Juliette. I was to consider her my patient.

Each morning, I placed my stethoscope against Juliette's chest. At first, I strained to hear the characteristic crunching of infected lung tissue; the sounds were distant, as if coming from another room. After three weeks, however, I could stand at the head of her bed and hear those coarse breath sounds unaided.

We gave Juliette more antibiotics, but their only effect was to exert just enough Darwinian pressure to allow the fittest bacteria to survive. As each day passed, more and more casualties of Juliette's immune system—slews of dead white blood cells—percolated from her breathing tube in the form of green and blood-tinged sputum. Eventually, toxins released from those hyper-resilient bacteria and from Juliette's immune system pushed her body into multisystem organ failure. First her respiratory system went, then her kidney and cardiovascular systems. She required a ventilator; she went on to require dialysis and a constant infusion of medications that would maintain her blood pressure at levels high enough to perfuse her brain.

Over the course of three weeks Juliette would become a human shell, and her life would be maintained by machines and medical professionals and the frightened medical student who kept vigil over her in the ICU.

Throughout Juliette's hospital course, Joseph, her husband of more than fifty years, managed to visit every day. It was not an easy feat. That winter was one of the worst in Chicago in recent memory, and there were no children or relatives to help Joseph get to our hospital. Joseph was easily over six feet tall and thin—what I imagined an elderly Ichabod Crane would look like had he lived in Chicago in the 1980s. He showed up at Juliette's bedside dressed in a black overcoat, hat, and gloves, smelling like the home of my sister's elderly piano teacher—a combination of mothballs and musty carpets. His translucent skin was stretched so tautly over his face and beaklike nose that I could see the tangle of fine blood vessels lying just beneath the surface and the S of the artery under his temples pulsating as he spoke. His eyes were blue, with crusts in the corners; at certain angles and in certain lighting, his irises shimmered. The first morning of Juliette's admission, he looked tired, having waited for hours in the crowded, noisy emergency room until Juliette was settled in the ICU.

Juliette and Joseph lived alone in an apartment just outside the city. Both junior high school teachers, they had met fifty-five years earlier when their homerooms were right next to each other. They spent most of that school year just smiling; but six months after Joseph summoned up the courage to ask Juliette out for dinner, they were married. When I asked Joseph about first meeting Juliette, he said that "she was the most beautiful woman in the world." I had occasionally heard fellow classmates sing such praises about their current girlfriends, and I usually laughed at the hyperbole. However, when I heard an eighty-five-year-old man married to the same woman for over half a century say it, I was silenced by the understatement.

Juliette and Joseph remained childless, but they were devoted to each other and to the city's public school system, retiring after putting in almost a hundred years combined. Slowly, over the course of time, they watched their contemporaries and their own siblings pass away until all that was left of their social circle was a distant nephew in another state and a stray friend here or there confined to a nursing home. With their health relatively intact, they settled into a quiet routine. After breakfast they took a morning walk. The rest of the day, until dinner, they read the newspaper, wrote social notes to their few surviving friends, and fussed over bills that arrived with the afternoon mail.

In the early morning of Juliette's admission to the hospital, Joseph noticed that his wife had become lethargic. She had developed a cough over the previous week and a fever the day before. That morning Joseph found that Juliette could not even answer his questions without falling asleep. Joseph called 911, and within an hour, his wife was diagnosed with a life-threatening pneumonia. The pneumonia that she had been harboring on a subclinical level all week had worsened markedly overnight, and she could no longer breathe well enough to sustain her body's oxygen levels. That difficulty breathing also prevented her from exhaling adequately, so she was unable to expel the carbon dioxide in her body. By the early morning the carbon dioxide had reached levels high enough to narcotize her brain.

The paramedics who arrived at their apartment placed a plastic oxygen mask over Juliette's face and rapidly moved her to a stretcher and then to the ambulance. As the ambulance drove away, lights flashing and sirens screaming into the morning darkness, Joseph was left to follow. Did he have enough cash for a taxi? Would the subways be running? Could he navigate his way through the city without her?

When Joseph finally arrived in the emergency room, a team of physicians surrounded Juliette. Her arterial blood gas—a measure of oxygenation in the arterial blood—was precariously low despite high levels of supplemental oxygen. Moreover, she was more and more somnolent from the high carbon dioxide blood levels and exhausted from trying to get enough air. As Joseph entered Juliette's room, he could see the physicians placing a tube into her mouth that would help her breathe but prevent her from speaking. Simultaneously they were administering a sedative to keep her from fighting the hard sensation of plastic in her throat.

Joseph moved quickly to Juliette's side and tried to hold her struggling hand. Of that moment Joseph only knew that his last words to his conscious wife were "I'm here, Juliette. I'm here." In response to those words, Joseph later told me, his wife fluttered her eyes and began biting on her breathing tube. That action, spied by emergency room personnel, brought Juliette more sedation to prevent her from clenching down on the breathing tube and asphyxiating herself. Juliette never regained consciousness.

In the early days of Juliette's nearly four-week stay, the medical intensive care unit team went over each aspect of her case in excruciating detail during our twice-daily rounds. We reviewed every laboratory result, we questioned every potential antibiotic change, we discussed every ventilator setting. The attending physician in charge of the ICU that month was a brash and brilliant young diagnostician who had eyes that twitched and darted about, the nervous tics of the hyper-intelligent. Members of his family—his sister and his brother—were also physicians at the hospital, and together with their legendary clinical skills, they formed a kind of dynastic hold on the medical center. While his sister and brother were known for their gentler touch, this attending reveled in his "tough guy" reputation with the trainees. After every presentation on rounds, he mercilessly interrogated students and residents, grilling them on the minutiae of each case and the research supporting different treatment options.

As Juliette's pneumonia became more resistant to our therapeutic maneuvers, however, the attending and the residents became less interested in the fine points of her case. And after three weeks I barely finished reciting my attempts at a plan for her care before the crowd huddled on rounds moved on to the next patient. One morning I quickly mentioned that I had seen some blood coming out of her nasogastric tube. The attending, already on his way to the next bed, stopped. He walked back over to me and picked up Juliette's tube to examine the dark red streaks. He surveyed her body, now bloated with illness. "Why don't you just wash her stomach out using that nasogastric tube, a syringe, and a bucket of cold saline?" he suggested.

I knew that procedure was part of the treatment for gastric bleeding, but I wanted him to say more. This newest change in Juliette's condition had to elicit some interest on the attending's part. After all, I had seen such cases before and knew that they sometimes required specialist intervention from a gastroenterologist or a surgeon. Some cases were even fatal.

"You're going to be a surgeon, aren't you?" he asked me. I nodded. "Then you can take care of it," he said, walking away and leaving me holding Juliette's bloody nasogastric tube. He winked at the other team members, or perhaps—as I convinced myself at that moment—his nervous twitch started up again. He continued rounds at the next bed and never again set foot in Juliette's room.

The nurses and I continued to roll Juliette over several times a day to clean the deepening, raw pressure sores on her back and buttocks. Oozing red flesh craters marked the areas where the pressure of her weight had caused the bones to wear through skin. Accompanied by the constant wheezing and hissing of the ventilator calliope next to her bed, we cleaned out Juliette's breathing tube and sucked out the mucus plugs in her lungs with a long, pliant catheter. We threaded that red rubber tube so far down her airway that it caused Juliette to go into fits of coughing, which in turn would launch her ventilator into its own refrain of whistles, cries, and flashing red lights. Although she was sedated, I remember Juliette wincing during these coughing spells, her torso arching up and her hands reaching frantically for the railings.

Occasionally, the nurses asked me to draw Juliette's blood, a task that became more difficult as her arms became swollen and veins scarred from the countless punctures. Once a single red drop fell from the syringe to my clogs. Because it had been so difficult to obtain, I cursed the loss of that precious microliter. That stain is still there on the clogs, which I still wear, almost as dark as it was that day.

Whenever I saw Joseph, I would wander over to him and try to make conversation. I wondered what he thought every time we asked him to step outside the room so we could take care of his wife. I wanted to know if he could hear the clanging alarms or the harsh, throaty cries coming through Juliette's breathing tube. I wanted to ask if he saw the piles of dirty linens bearing the cloying smell of the hospital's cleaning agents along with his wife's sweat and other body fluids. I wanted to apologize for hurting his wife every time he stepped outside her room at my request, to ask him if he was angry that the only people he ever talked to were the nurses and the medical student, and to tell him that it wasn't just that there were a lot of sick people who needed care in the ICU, but that the doctors had lost interest in a case that could have only one outcome.

While I desperately wanted the authority of my attending so that I could relay to Joseph all that I knew, I felt relieved not to be responsible for telling him that his wife was dying. When I actually did approach Joseph, I squeezed all those thoughts behind my best compassionate expression and asked him if he wanted a glass of water or a cup of coffee. We both knew that as the lowest member on the medical totem pole, I could offer little more. Then I tried to fill the emptiness of our exchange with chatter about the weather or the latest headlines.

I worried about Joseph. He always came alone, and at times he seemed like little more than a wraith that the infamous Chicago wind had blown in. From a seat in the nursing station across from Juliette's bed, I surreptitiously watched him visiting his unconscious wife. More and more Joseph fell asleep at his wife's bedside, his head against the safety railing of the bed and his hand still locked on hers. He stopped noticing when I walked up to Juliette's bed and even when I tried to make conversation. His cheeks began to appear unevenly shaven, and occasionally, a white rim of dried toothpaste lined his thin, chapped lips. Joseph's smell changed, too; there was the faint odor of urine now laced in with the mothballs and musty carpets.

On the night Juliette died, Chicago was buried by one of the worst snowstorms of the decade. One of the senior residents called Joseph to tell him that his wife was unlikely to make it through the night. I know Joseph struggled to get to our unit. I know because the radio kept announcing that the salt shortage would prevent Chicago streets from getting plowed until the morning. Having been stuck at the hospital the previous night on call, I was busy trying to figure out how to make one change of clothes last several days.

I sat at the nursing station directly in front of Juliette's bed and stared at her monitors. The heartbeats began to slow, and the once regular waveforms took on a jagged irregularity, images of the last contractions of life. I knew that Joseph did not have much time to get to Juliette. Across from her bed, the nurses and I quietly waited for the permanent pause that would signal to us to pronounce her death and to prepare Juliette's body for the morgue.

When Joseph arrived, he pulled up his usual chair and took off his dark hat, gloves, and coat. He sat down, maneuvered his hand between the metal safety railings, and held Juliette's hand between his cold fingers. He whispered to her and bent his aged head over hers. A nurse switched off the erratically beeping cardiac monitor in

Juliette's room and gently closed the curtains around the two of them.

Joseph finally emerged from the room with his coat in hand. From the monitors at the nursing station, I knew that Juliette's heart had finally stopped. I approached Joseph, asking him if he would be all right going back out into the snow. I did not know what else to say. There was no one else there to talk to him; the residents and attendings had disappeared. Joseph shook his head at my offer of help and walked out of the ICU.

Fifteen years later, I can still see that tall, ghostly figure leaving the unit. The halls are dark and empty, and the walls shimmer with reflections from the windows of snow falling quietly onto the Chicago streets.

Is it possible to change the way physicians care for the dying? During the mid-1990s, a group of researchers tried to answer that question in a pivotal study of American end-of-life care. With millions of dollars in funding, the SUPPORT study (Study to Understand Prognoses and Preferences for Outcomes and Risks of Treatments) first assessed the quality of care provided by hundreds of physicians and health care workers to thousands of patients with life-threatening diagnoses.

The initial findings were dismal. A large proportion of terminal patients spent their last days in an intensive care unit. A majority of physicians had no idea what their patients wanted in terms of resuscitation; and, according to family members, fully half of hospitalized patients who remained conscious at the end of life complained of moderate or severe pain at least half the time.

With these initial results in hand, the SUPPORT researchers discussed possible ways to respond to what seemed to be deficiencies in communication and information. They decided to implement the most intensive interventions possible. They hired specially trained nurses; these nurses talked to the patients and their families about their diagnoses, their understanding of prognoses, and their preferences regarding treatment. The nurses then communicated regularly with the patients' physicians and with the hospital staff. The researchers also created frequent reports based on a sophisticated computer model of survival prognosis and on interviews with patients and their families, and they inserted these reports into patient charts.

The results of these Herculean interventions were completely unexpected: after two years of active intervention, the SUPPORT researchers found *no* notable improvements. Terminal patients in the last six months of their lives still received aggressive treatment, and many of them were in the intensive care unit. A high percentage of these patients continued to complain of moderate to severe pain at the end of their lives; and a large number of physicians still had no idea of their patients' final wishes regarding cardiopulmonary resuscitation and artificial life support.

Why did all these efforts to improve the situation fail so miserably?

Experts in end-of-life care have offered several possible explanations. One may be that physicians cannot bear to undermine a patient's optimism and will continue aggressive therapy in order to maintain a glimmer of hope. Another reason may be the increased specialization of our medical system; since dying patients are often under the care of myriad specialists, no single physician is ultimately responsible for facilitating end-of-life choices. These terminal patients and the difficult associated discussions end up being punted to and fro between doctors until the topic either is forgotten or becomes irrelevant.

There may be financial or legal reasons. Prolonged

care is associated with monetary gain for some doctors. More often, however, physicians will continue aggressive care because they fear litigation, sometimes irrationally so. They may be concerned that the courts will construe any other approach to care as inadequately attentive or as hastening death. They may hesitate to administer adequate pain medications, believing that prescriptions for large doses of narcotics will be interpreted as irresponsible or even criminal.

Patients, too, may be in part responsible for this depressing situation, since they may hesitate to be assertive, fearing potential negative repercussions from their doctors. Other patients may follow their own cultural beliefs, believe that they are being prejudicially refused "full court press" efforts, or try to preserve their outward dignity by ignoring the suggestions of those around them to inform physicians of their wishes. A significant number of patients also deny life-threatening illnesses; as many as 10 percent of patients hospitalized with advanced cancer are in severe denial, while an additional 18 percent exhibit moderate levels of denial. While this coping mechanism can sometimes be helpful for dying patients, for others denial results in unrealistic expectations and the failure to make all the necessary arrangements for the end of life. It may also be a marker for depression.

Whatever the factors contributing to the study's abysmal results, it is clear that the physicians in the study continued to work from within their own psychological framework regardless of outside efforts to improve communication. Despite the researchers' efforts, the doctors did not change. Dying patients continued to be a profound source of unease that physicians avoided or ignored.

That uneasiness is not so foreign to many of us, physician or not. After all, most people would rather not think about death even occasionally, let alone deal with it head-on day after day. However, since all of us will die, the role of the physician, frequently the guardian of those last days, is paramount. What is most significant then about the results from the SUPPORT study is not the disheartening state of dying in America. It is how we physicians have lost insight into our own dysfunctional anxiety and how that anxiety has in turn become immortalized within our medical system.

These deeply entrenched behaviors that we physicians embrace are not like the surgical gloves that we can learn to slide on and snap off. They are present even before we decide to become doctors and are ingrained by invisible yet powerful professional values until our last days of practice. Despite our best efforts to improve, our apprenticeship system continues to produce doctors who are unable to care humanely for the dying. The attitudes we physicians have toward death become reinforced each and every time we learn from our attendings and then go on to teach others.

As the clinical aphorism goes, "See one, do one, teach one."

Rather than setting out to improve treatment, as we do with diseases, we continue to treat dying as ineffectively as our professional forefathers. This deeply rooted angst about death thus replicates itself over and over again like some tragic hereditary disease. And like those terrible genetic disorders, this one, too, gets passed unknowingly from one generation to another.

I first met Kay in my second year of residency. At the time, Kay was in her late sixties and worked as a receptionist in the operating room. Born into an upper-middle-class

Boston family, Kay married soon after college and had two sons. In her mid-thirties, she started a catering business in southwestern Massachusetts that eventually became, as she advertised, the "presence that adds elegance" to every wedding, graduation, retirement, and business affair in the region.

Pictures of Kay from her youth show a tall, slender woman with Katharine Hepburn cheekbones and intense eyes. In her form-fitting dresses, white gloves, and hats, she looked like the women in the black-and-white fashion photos of the 1950s. Although she still had that larger-than-life aura by the time we met, Kay hardly looked like the old pictures. In her early fifties, she had developed a gambling and drinking habit so severe that she lost her business, marriage, and self-respect all within five years. The Kay I knew wore sweatpants and baggy holiday-themed sweaters on her six-foot frame, never wore makeup, rarely wore jewelry, and lived in a small studio apartment packed with old Christmas cards, photos, and Weight Watchers frozen meal trays. Her only vice now was smoking. Other than her work for the operating room and her regular 12-step meetings, the one thing that filled Kay's life was her AIDS patients.

Kay's eldest son, her beloved Matthew, had died of AIDS a few years after Kay left rehabilitation. The experience of watching Matthew die drove Kay to spend countless hours working with those dying from AIDS. Sometimes I wondered if Kay was compelled to love others because she had not been able to love her own son during those years consumed by gambling and drinking. Whatever her motivation, Kay became a well-known figure in the New Haven AIDS community, a source of unquestioning comfort and love when families refused to support dying relatives because of their own notions of respectability and shame.

In my last two years of residency I moved to an apartment across the hall from Kay. Some evenings, tired from the forty-hour shifts in the hospital, I wandered over to Kay's and listened to her stories about Matthew and about the AIDS patients. There was apartment-bound John, whose father shunned him and who needed his laundry done. There was Linda, who did not have the means to get to her doctors' appointments to care for her disease. There was Sandra, who remained estranged from her family despite being weeks away from death.

Kay was always there for them.

And it seemed she was there for almost everyone else, including me, her surgical resident neighbor who frequently came over to complain about work and boyfriends. One evening Kay knocked at my door, asking for my professional help. On the eighth floor of our apartment building, two elderly brothers, both Catholic priests, had developed two separate surgical problems—an inguinal hernia and a diabetic foot ulcer. Kay, who had grown up in their parish in Boston, had been dispensing their pills and preparing them for their winter trip to Florida. She wanted me to check one priest's groin and the other's feet. For the next four weeks, Kay made sure that during my evenings off, I spent a few hours with Father Bill and Father John, checking their wounds, massaging their feet, and helping her get them in and out of bed.

When I left New Haven to go to Los Angeles for subspecialty fellowship training, I kept in touch with Kay through letters. In truth, Kay wrote most of the letters; work was the busiest it had ever been, and I hardly had time to sleep. I had only one four-day vacation that first year, and I was drawn back to New Haven to visit Kay. She had just gotten a new car, a used white Cadillac that she had bought at a particularly good price, and she was thrilled. She took me outside to admire it, and afterward we had tea in her cramped quarters. Before I left, we took pictures. In those photos, Kay is towering over me, her oversized hyperopic glasses emphasizing her large brown eyes. I remember that it was during the Christmas season because ornaments are hanging on the window in the background. She is wearing a white sweatshirt with a red AIDS ribbon in the center that forms the O for the word "Hope." Her turtleneck is red and her pants are white. White is the color of death in Chinese culture; I remember her laughing when I told her she probably should not wear this outfit to take care of her AIDS patients. In the picture, I am smiling, and she is wiping her tears away with her left hand. She looks robust and healthy.

Six months later, I received a letter from Kay. She wrote that she had developed cancer in her liver. *Would you know anything about it?* She knew that I was specializing in liver surgery and thought I might be able to help her out. I called to ask for copies of her X-rays and her biopsy report. Kay was upbeat on the phone. "Oh, it's nothing I can't handle," she said. "Besides, I have my patients to take care of."

The biopsy of Kay's liver revealed adenocarcinoma from an unknown primary site; the malignant tumor had already spread to her liver. In the same envelope with the biopsy report I found copies of Kay's CAT scan. Holding the pictures up to the light, I saw a horrifying image. On the scan the tumors looked like black holes within the body of Kay's liver; every segment of her liver was riddled, like a corpse after a gangland shooting. Kay could not survive more than a few months. I took her reports and films for review by experts in my medical center, and they agreed with my dire prediction. Chemotherapy would be Kay's only option, but the chances of response would be exceedingly slim. I called Kay to convey this message to her. She still sounded optimistic on the phone. Her doctors in New Haven had said the same thing, and she was planning on starting chemotherapy the following week.

I did not call Kay again.

One evening six months later, a former residency colleague named Carla left a message on my voice mail. She also knew Kay well. Kay was now in hospice and asked about me often. Carla said she wanted to pass on the message from Kay. I wept but did not call Kay.

A month later, Carla called again. This time I answered the phone. "Kay is dying," Carla said, as if I might not have known Kay's prognosis. "She doesn't have long." I told Carla that work had been busy but I had been meaning to call. I promised to call the next day.

A week went by. Every time I saw a terminal patient at work, I thought of Kay. In fact, I thought of her almost constantly that week but could not bring myself to call. Finally, one afternoon, sitting alone in my office, I found a letter that Kay had written a year prior, before she knew about her cancer. She ended it as she ended all her letters to me. Her handwriting was, like Kay, big and loopy. *I pray for you, Pauline. I pray that the year will be more gentle for you. Love, Kay XXOO.*

I picked up my phone and called Kay. Her voice on the phone was ecstatic. She forgave me quickly for not calling. "I know you are busy," she said. When I asked her how she was doing, she replied that she had some pain, but the people in hospice had been so kind to her, and one of her favorite priests, Father George, visited her regularly. "I probably have a week left," she said to me on the phone, so she was happy to have heard my voice. "I keep thinking, Pauline, that I am finally going to be with my Matthew." Kay must have heard my voice wavering because she then said, "I'm not in pain, Pauline. I'm really very comfortable."

A couple of months later I received a letter from Kay's

other son, Tom. Kay did die a week after our phone conversation, pain-free and peaceful. Tom thanked me for being his mother's friend and wrote about how much our friendship had meant to Kay. I looked at the program from her memorial service, enclosed in the envelope. I recognized the prayer within as one of her favorites, and above it there was a picture of Kay, smiling and as I remembered her. I suddenly felt as if my heart had disappeared out of my chest, leaving a large empty hole that even my lungs could not fill. I wanted to cry, but instead stashed the letter into a far corner of my desk drawer.

Through my training, I had a recurring dream. I am wandering in a large building, looking for a room in which to settle. The building is dark, nearly windowless, and every room I walk into is either too small or too large. Finally, I find one that seems just right except that it has a window with its curtains parted slightly. At first I need to squint and cover my eyes; I have been in the dark for so long that even this small amount of light hurts.

I am not sure I want this room. Eventually, though, my eyes adjust to the light and I walk toward the window, mesmerized by the sun's warmth against my face. I want to draw the curtains open, look out, and let the sunlight fill the entire room. But then I wake up.

My dying patients and their families affected my life so deeply that they inhabited my dreams for years, even if in the most symbolic of forms. They were the very human reminders of the complexity of my profession, and they were the unexpected findings of my training.

One of the tenets of surgical training is that performing an operation over and over again makes the steps become second nature. But while the steps create an essential framework, the unforeseen complications encountered during repeated practice become our greatest challenges. Dealing with the contents of a burst appendix, working through the matted intestines of a scarred belly, or stemming the life-threatening torrential bleeding in a cirrhotic patient—these are the experiences that bring true wisdom and finesse to our surgical skills.

Becoming a doctor is no different. Just as with surgery, my peers and I practiced *being* doctors by caring for patients. But what perturbed my well-practiced routines were the terminal patients, the grieving families, and even the dead themselves. I had never expected to deal with the dying so intimately or to face mortality so directly.

Like the unforeseen complications in the operating room, these unexpected findings of my profession, perhaps more than anything else, challenged and then shaped the surgeon I would become.

II

PRACTICE

Chapter 4

THE INFORMAL CURRICULUM

For over two years I dreaded scrubbing my hands. Just starting was overwhelming; each time I reached above the operating room sinks to take one of those pre-packaged, pre-soaped scrub brushes, dozens more would tumble forth, hurling themselves at me like lemmings falling into the sea. The actual scrubbing, a ten-minute procedure required before the first operation of the day, was even more daunting: "Twenty swipes per surface over thirty seconds," "one minute for each set of fingers," "one minute on the back of the hand," "one minute on the palms," and "one minute on each side of each arm to just the elbows."

Every morning I stood there nearly paralyzed. I had

convinced myself that poor scrub technique would allow the scheming, hyper-reproductive bacteria on my arms to hop onto the unsuspecting patient and wreak havoc. Moreover, I dreaded my own fate in such cases. A single error at the sink erased any hope that day of my being a "promising" or even "helpful" student; rather, I became "the contaminated medical student." And after all my years of schooling *that* was a failure of the highest order. In front of everyone—attending surgeons, residents, anesthesiologists, nurses, OR technicians, even the sleeping patient—the nurses would hustle me back to the sink, their admonition to "Go back and wash your hands again" breaking the hallowed silence. The half a dozen times that happened, my shame was almost too much to bear.

Eventually, after an internship's worth of struggles at the sink, scrubbing up became second nature. With eyes closed, I could smoothly pivot my left knee and start up a gentle rush of water from the hands-free faucet. I came to favor a certain brand of soap and the brushes with the saffron-colored sponge and soft bristles. After I'd worked all night and then rushed through patient rounds in the early morning, those ten minutes in front of the sink provided a comfortable respite, a few meditative moments in an otherwise frenetic day.

Throughout the years I barely varied the way I scrubbed. Even in the dead of New England winters when the windchill factor dipped, I scrubbed as I had learned as a medical student. I would turn on the water, soak my arms, and move the brush back and forth, stirring up white, silky foam over every square millimeter of skin. And as I scrubbed I would look above the sink and over the transom into the OR. I would see my patient moving over from gurney to operating room table and the anesthesiologists deliberately mixing their concoctions for sleep.

Sometimes in those minutes I would feel a burn from the sharp points of the brush, but the feeling would pass as I moved to another part of my arm and became mesmerized again by the circular scrubbing motions.

After ten minutes I would drop the brush into the wastebasket and pass my arms under the stream of warm water. Only then, after the clinging soapsuds had fallen away into the sink, would I again feel the sting. Amid the glistening cleanness of my skin, I would notice the back of my chapped hands and how there now were, after my ritual ablution, jagged red lines meandering across my flesh.

I spent all of my young adulthood learning to be a doctor. After medical school, there were five years of general surgery internship and residency, interrupted by two years of cancer research and training, all of which was topped off with a final two years of transplantation and liver surgery subspecialization. There were nine years in all, nine years spent living clinical surgery.

People, particularly medical students about to decide on specialties, have asked me what it was like to spend so many years in training. I used to answer that clinical training was like the priesthood; your chosen field was a "calling," and that calling required sequestering yourself away from the world for a few years. I liked the romanticism of that response, and for almost all nine years, I believed it. After all, attending to the ill was about as noble a calling as one could have.

I was in my ninth year when that changed. I had been up all night because of a difficult transplant; specifically, the recipient patient's hepatic artery kept shredding. The hepatic artery is the main conduit of oxygenated blood in a transplanted liver, and for that reason, this reconstruction—attaching the new artery to the recipient's artery—is one of the most important predictors of a patient's outcome. Done perfectly, it allows patients to recover within a week and come back to your clinic a month later looking as if you had never laid hands on them. Done imperfectly, it causes the organ to fail, sending patients spiraling downward back into liver failure and possibly death. There are few such clear-cut consequences in medicine.

That night every stitch ate away at the recipient's artery, leaving the stump shorter and more ragged each time we tried. Three attempts later, we finally got the perfect, pulsating connection. It was 4:00 a.m.

At 4:30, after the operation was essentially done, the attending surgeon left my close friend Susan, also a surgical fellow, and me to finish closing up the patient's skin. Together she and I had been up for over forty-eight hours. To hurry us along and prevent us from falling over, the sympathetic nurses had put "closing music"—pulsating dance club music—on the sound system. The muscles in my hands ached from operating, and the soles of my feet throbbed. Over the years I had learned that these were my cardinal signs of exhaustion.

When the last stitch was finally in, Susan looked up at me. Even covered with a surgical mask and the bug-eyed surgical loupe glasses, she exuded fatigue. Our chatty conversation had stopped a couple of hours ago—all we wanted to do now was go home to sleep—so I was surprised when she began talking again.

"Is this what training is all about?" Susan asked me. She took a sterile wet cloth and wiped off the blood from the patient's skin before laying down the dressing. Susan continued, not waiting for my answer. "You or me—would we have kept redoing that hepatic artery?" She laughed, then said, "I kept praying each time that it would work so that I could go to bed." I did not reply, but my silence was confirmation enough. "But the boss," Susan continued, referring to our mentor, "he wouldn't let it go."

We both stepped back from the table and stripped off our operating gowns and gloves. With a decade and a half of training between us, neither of us was willing to concede—exhausted or not—that we had gone through all of that for naught.

"Maybe training is doing the thing right so many times over," Susan said at last, "that you eventually cannot accept anything else." She paused, then added, "Even if you're totally exhausted."

I thought about Susan's words the next day. I thought about them six months later when I finished my training. When I finally began doing those hepatic arteries on my own, I realized that she was right. No matter how exhausted I was—or angry or happy or busy—when it came down to that reconstruction, everything disappeared from my mind except for the simple, perfect tension-bearing stitches I had to sew around that pencil-thin artery.

And because we had talked about it, I began noticing that Susan's observation held true beyond the hepatic artery. There were other procedures I had practiced so many times through the years that they had become as much a part of me as brushing my teeth at night.

After nine years of clinical training, I found it hard to conceive of doing these clinical tasks any differently. In fact, I believed there was no other way, because these rituals were what assured the quality of my practice. They were what made me a good doctor.

.   .   .

Most doctors spend their lives trying to be good at what they do; we want our patients to love us, our colleagues to respect us, and our families and communities to beam with pride. But all of our future professional accomplishments are premised on our training. We begin with an almost blind trust in that training, voluntarily devoting most or all of our young adult lives and suppressing outside interests with the belief that in the end we will come out right.

In the process hospitals become our makeshift homes, and the attending physicians, fellow residents, and nurses become our surrogate families. Twice a year, as a resident, I gave tours of the hospital to medical students applying for the residency program. I always said the same thing as we passed by the cafeteria or the cluttered on-call rooms shared by a half dozen residents. "This is my kitchen," I would say. "That is my bedroom." The medical students would always giggle, but in a year's time as interns they would give a new set of applicants the same tour.

Eventually, like children, we learn to embrace the values of our new family. There is, for example, a strong oral tradition in residencies. Older residents exchange stories with new initiates, passing the culture down through successive generations in the trenches of training. Like fables, these anecdotes are infused with the values of the profession. During the early years of my training, I gobbled up these tales; I was as eager to learn them as to create some common ground with the other residents. They restructured my view of the hospital microcosm, and I found ways in which my own beginning clinical experiences validated their unshakable veracity.

Medical sociologists have long understood that clinical training involves more than just learning about diseases and therapy. Through what they have termed as the "informal" or "hidden" curriculum of medical training, young doctors are assimilated into a medical culture that espouses certain norms of behavior and emotion. Slang terms, subtle gestures, unspoken decisions, and the canon of clinical fables all feed into this value system. In absorbing the lessons of the hidden curriculum, young doctors cease being laypeople and learn to become doctors. And among the most cherished lessons are those concerning the innate goodness of rituals.

With all the vagaries of human illness and emotion in the clinical world, it is hardly surprising that doctors focus so much on rituals. For most people, even in daily life, the oft-repeated patterns of rituals create a comfortable and reassuring scaffolding. Rituals like Sunday dinners, bedtime stories, and the morning coffee and newspaper provide us with predictable security. On the one hand we depend on them to get through the day and week; on the other hand they allow us to make sense of our individual place in the world by representing those values we believe most important.

Medical students and residents spend the majority of their training practicing clinical rituals variously called "procedures," "protocols," and "algorithms." When we see patients in the clinics, we perform a history and physical exam, and we go through a prescribed checklist of questions that every physician in the country has memorized. Our admission orders and discharge orders have standardized patterns that we all know by heart. Our operating atlases list steps for each procedure. Even the government acknowledges the overarching importance of rituals in clinical practice by grouping diagnoses and parceling out financial reimbursements accordingly.

Implicit in all of these rituals is the belief that was expressed by my friend Susan. We believe that our training will teach us the rituals and that they in turn will allow us to rise above human fallibility.

And it is not only physicians who find comfort in this belief. Patients see the profusion of standardized protocols and procedures as a reliable system of checks and balances. Any one of us who has sat on an examining table covered by a flimsy hospital gown or who has waited to fall asleep on the operating table surrounded by sharp instruments probably finds such attention to details reassuring.

However, learning any of these rituals, even one as relatively straightforward as scrubbing, can be daunting to the medical student or resident. And the more complicated rituals, like learning to open someone's belly or resuscitating the mangled trauma victim or transplanting a liver, are downright dizzying and require you to put your innate responses on hold in order to perfect the dozens of discrete steps.

Eventually, though, through years of practice, you find that you stop wincing when you see the gleaming, sharp blade meet skin and draw bright blood. You no longer feel the pit in your stomach when the burn victim, reeking of charred flesh, rolls into the emergency room. And while the magic of healing another person never fades, you find yourself forgetting, as you focus on getting through the operation or the resuscitation or even the simplest exam, about the patient who is now in your hands. Instead, the person before you becomes yet another case in your clinical experience, and all you can concentrate on is getting through your work without making a mistake. The more difficult the case, the deeper you draw upon your memory banks, cashing in on the dozens of times you have done the same ritual before. You want nothing more than to perform all the steps perfectly and to leave your patient, by virtue of your meticulous attention to ritual, with life force completely intact.

· · ·

Relying on rituals was never more important than when I was caring for a child in need of a liver transplant. Child-sized donor organs are rare, so pediatric patients with hepatic failure must wait even as the liver disease exhausts their precious few physiologic reserves. Often comatose, they lie in beds meant for adults, hemmed in by a bevy of machines that whirr, whistle, and beep over their every movement, mechanical nannies who cannot stop clucking. Why, I asked myself each time I stood at the foot of these hellish arrangements, have these children ended up so different from those on the playground down the street?

In my second year of transplant training, two-year-old Michael spent a week waiting in our intensive care unit. His father, a hulking man with hands as large as my head, and his mother, a sinewy, athletic-looking woman, sat constantly at their son's bedside. Michael's father kept telling me about the recurring image he had of his son. "He just learned to dance a couple of weeks ago. He would stand by the speakers, bopping up and down with that smile on his face." The few pictures taped up around Michael's bed showed a chortling toddler with dimples so deep they seemed to anchor his cheeks into a permanent smile.

My younger brother has the same dimples.

Michael had developed acute liver failure after what was thought to be an unremarkable viral illness. "He usually would be running from the moment he woke up, but he just kept wanting to lie down and be held," Michael's mother said. After a few days she noticed that the whites of Michael's eyes had turned yellow. "That was when," she said, "I got this horrible sinking feeling in my stomach."

When Michael had probably no more than a day to live, we received news that a liver was available for him. I had already performed almost fifty other transplant organ procurements by the time I went out to get that liver for Michael, and the operation, with its multitude of steps and enmeshed decision trees, had become pretty routine. But the organs and vessels of children, whether donors or recipients, are so much smaller than an adult's that any slightly imperfect stitch or sloppily placed cut can be disastrous.

That night I hardly noticed the glittering Los Angeles city lights as we flew by helicopter down the Pacific coast. By the time we arrived at the hospital's operating rooms, the nurses had prepared the donor; there was only a strip of flesh extending from the base of the neck to the pubic bone exposed among the layers of operative drapes. I remember making the incision down that narrow path, my mind straining over the miniaturization. I felt as if I had been dropped into a diminutive china shop and that any inadvertent twist of my wrists would cause everything to shatter. I kept asking for smaller, finer, sharper dissecting scissors, and my neck ached as I struggled to see every detail. My scalp became warm and itchy under the hot OR heating lamps.

When we finally removed the liver, a plum-colored organ with surfaces as soft as velvet, I wanted only to close up as quickly as possible. I kept thinking about hurrying back to Michael.

With thick black sutures I lashed together the edges of the gaping incision. After finishing I nearly tripped over wiring on the floor as I rushed to leave the OR. "You look awfully awake for this time of the night," one of the nurses commented as I peeled off my bloodied OR gown and stuffed it into the trash bin. I felt relieved and triumphant.

Just before leaving, however, I stopped in the operating room once more to pick up a few documents. By now the nurses had removed the drapes from the body, and I saw a small boy lying naked on the table.

The sight of that child, cold and dead under the bright lights, stunned me. I had just had my hands wrist-deep in his belly, but I had never noticed the grass stains on those knobby knees or the face splattered with orange freckles or the spiky red halo of hair.

A large red tire-patterned abrasion covered the side of his chest, interrupted by several deeply embedded flecks of gravel. His mother, the nurses told me, had been unloading groceries from the car when the boy's six-year-old sister climbed into the driver's seat and shifted out of park. The boy fell in the path of the front wheels. By the time his mother heard his sister's screams, the boy was breathing irregularly, his upper chest pressed into the gravel driveway by the weight of the car.

I saw the long incision and the black stitches I had left. While the rest of his body still bore traces of baby fat—chubby, short fingers and rocker feet—his abdomen, which should have been the most soft and round and full, sank down and looked like the emptied cavity it now was.

I stood agape. My own chest felt empty and my head throbbed. I began to wonder what ran through his mother's mind when she came back out of the house and saw him. I wondered how her shrieks and cries rang through the neighborhood and what the little boy's sister thought when she saw her mother wailing and her brother unresponsive. I wanted for a moment to rip apart those black sutures, to put the organs back, and to shake the dead boy back to consciousness. I wanted to hold his mother, now long gone from the hospital, and apologize that with all my instruments and maneuvers and training I could not roll back time.

On the helicopter ride back along the coast, I forgot

about this favorite part of early morning procurements. I did not notice the rising sun reflected in the waves of the Pacific, the dolphins romping below, or the towering southern California bluffs. I even forgot for a moment about Michael. Instead, all I could think about, all I could see, were the small organs in the cooler next to me and the child I had left behind.

There is an oft-repeated aphorism in clinical medicine: every treatment is a double-edged sword. With every beneficial medication, there are adverse side effects. For every curative surgical procedure, there are complications.

Our rituals are no different. At the same time that they protect us from doing the wrong thing, their protective logic can shield us from fully shouldering responsibility. It is a powerful, upside-down form of self-defense for doctors: I did everything the right way, so I could not possibly have made a mistake.

It is precisely when that responsibility is largest— encompassing a powerful human emotion or even life itself—that concentrating on the ritual becomes our professional method of coping. The rituals allow us to evade death, literally and figuratively. We can spend as little time as possible with dying patients, concentrating instead on the "treatment algorithm" for their "disease process." We can never personalize our language or even mention the word "dying" in our conversations; we can instead discuss these cases in the context of objective data. In the hidden curriculum of medicine, younger doctors intuit that the end-stage cases are somehow less important than the failed ritual, and older doctors find comfort in the failed ritual's power to exonerate the individual.

These lessons are so powerful that even students who have learned about end-of-life care during their first two years of medical school are rapidly "untaught" once they enter the clinical realm.

Along the way, then, we learn not only to avoid but also to define death as the result of errors, imperfect technique, and poor judgment. Death is no longer a natural event but a ritual gone awry.

Two leaders in end-of-life care, Dr. Susan Block and Dr. J. Andrew Billings, have studied the complicated relationship between the informal curriculum and how young doctors eventually approach the care of the dying. Contrary to the unspoken lessons in many hospitals, Block and Billings believe that end-of-life care may be the ideal training ground for young doctors. They write:

> So long as appropriate emotional support is provided for learners, the immediacy and rawness of the emotions surrounding death for patients, families, and physicians can allow learning to take place at a deep level. Caring for the dying can also help young physicians learn to tolerate a degree of intimacy and personal engagement that other aspects of medical training may subvert and undermine.

By evading death, we miss one of the best opportunities for us to learn how "to doctor," because dealing with the dying allows us to nurture our best humanistic tendencies.

But taking hold of those opportunities requires changing the informal curriculum, and that is an enormous task.

By its very nature, the informal curriculum defies definition while permeating every aspect of a young physician's life. And even though nearly every medical school in the country has added formal courses on end-of-life care, changing that informal network of values and lessons requires even more profound reforms. For medical educators, it means being willing to, as medical sociologist F. W. Hafferty has written, "assess just what messages are being created by and within the very structures they have developed and are responsible for." Reforming the informal curriculum requires fundamental changes in the policies and values set forth by professional institutions and academic medical centers.

There have been a few small but significant changes in the last decade. National organizations that set the requirements of medical education and of physician certification now require exposure to and knowledge of palliative care. And while these requirements do not necessarily ensure adequate training in these skills, they are important value statements. In the last five years the American College of Surgeons, the largest professional group of surgeons, created a task force devoted to palliative care. Part of their goal was to look into the education of surgical residents. Tapping into the experiences of other specialties, the surgeons' task force began enrolling residents from different surgical programs into a palliative care course, excusing these trainees from their usually fixed work demands. Within one year, thirty-two surgical residency programs had been enrolled, and the residents who took the course reported greater comfort and confidence in dealing with patients at the end of life. These changes in attitude persisted six to eight months later when the residents were reevaluated. It appeared that this course and the importance placed on it had had a significant and lasting effect.

. . .

One winter, suffering from cracked, chapped skin once again, I decided to look into the research on scrubbing techniques. I had always been sort of a football player about my time at the operating room sinks—I believed in doing it until it hurt. I was never sure, however, that my approach to the ten-minute scrub stood up to any kind of scientific examination.

I discovered guidelines published in 2002 by the Centers for Disease Control for "hand hygiene in the health care setting." The authors of the report, after reviewing all the available research, found that scrubbing for five minutes reduced hand bacterial counts as effectively as ten minutes. Soft disposable sponges were as effective as hard, bristly brushes, and scrubbing with no brush at all could be sufficient if one used the right soap preparation.

The way I calculated it, then, over the course of more than a decade of scrubbing, I had spent close to an entire week's worth of time—seven days and nights—sudsing up for no reason at all.

The ten-minute scrub was one of the earliest rituals I had learned, and I thought that it was essential in surgical antisepsis, a crucial step in preventing my patients from developing debilitating postoperative infections. I had believed that my dedication to this operating room rite made me a good and responsible surgeon, but the research contradicted that belief. Suddenly my blind trust in the practice seemed almost foolish.

While many of the rituals we practice in medicine are structured attempts to deliver uniform quality care, our excessive devotion to them can obscure other important issues, such as patient and physician emotions. And although the current trend is to embrace evidence-based medicine—that is, clinical practice based on thoughtful, well-structured research—we still easily slip back into familiar routines when it comes to end-of-life care. As the SUPPORT study showed, even with the most extensive of efforts we will resort to old rituals that provide opportunities to flee from the dying.

As difficult as it sometimes seems to me, I have to believe that it is possible to practice our professional rituals while acknowledging their limitations. Practiced blindly, these rituals handicap us and foster a false sense of infallibility; practiced humanely, they can open the realm of healing. I know that because I have been witness to physicians who, through even the smallest alterations, changed rituals in the most dramatic of ways.

When a patient is dying in the intensive care unit, the protocol is always the same. Door or curtains are closed around the patient and family, the nurse turns off the monitors so the family does not have to hear the cardiac monitor go flatline, and physicians scatter in order to give the family some privacy.

I spent countless hours making myself scarce while waiting for patients to die. Sometimes the deaths took an hour, sometimes an entire afternoon. I lingered around the ICU computers, busying myself with test results. I looked in on other patients who were in the ICU. Mostly I fidgeted at the nursing station, unsure of when to go away and when to stay.

Eventually I would catch sight of family members coming out, limp tissues crushed in their fists. If they stood there long enough, and if the nurses' station monitors showed no more breathing or heartbeats, I knew it was all over. After the last family member had appeared and the appointed family spokesperson had heard my spiel on "what to do next," I went behind the curtains. There, alone with the deceased, I pronounced the patient officially dead in three steps and filled out the requisite paperwork.

One patient's death was different. He was a retired businessman whose colon cancer had spread to his liver and lungs. It was 4:00 a.m. when the man's heart began to fail and I telephoned my attending surgeon at home.

Within a half hour the surgeon arrived, his skin bearing the telltale lines of bedsheets. Soon afterward the patient's wife appeared at the entrance of the ICU. She was of average height and build, with sparkling diamond studs in her ears and long gray hair that she always wore swept up in a twist. I had talked with her many times about her teaching at a nearby high school, about their thirty-year marriage, and about the fact that she knew that her husband did not have long to live. Every afternoon I would see her at her husband's bedside, sitting erect and holding his hand or reading him a book or sharing a newspaper. She would jump up to greet me and then ask me to step outside the room for a moment. In the hallway she would ask me when her husband could leave the hospital to die at home.

She stopped asking when he became comatose and was transferred to the ICU.

The woman now stood stiffly by the unit secretary's desk, her eyes red and puffy and her lips drawn tightly closed. I tried to smile, not sure how to greet a woman who was about to watch her lifelong partner die. All I could think of saying was "I'm sorry." She nodded in response and looked over toward her husband's room.

I felt myself pulling away. I could not convince myself that the woman would be happier alone with her dying husband. But there was little I could do to stop; it was as if the familiar ritual had already been set in motion. I took a step back and fell hard against a chair, having tripped over my own feet.

My attending surgeon took the woman's hand and quietly explained what was happening. Her mouth opened and she began sobbing. He gently led her to the room, where I saw her jerk forward, crumpling in front of her husband's bed. The surgeon then walked back toward me, but instead of leaving the woman in the room alone, he closed the curtains around the three of them.

I hung back for a few minutes but became curious when the surgeon did not step out. What was he doing in there? Why didn't he leave her, as we always did?

I peeked in. Inside, the woman was still sobbing, but she was standing with her hand in her husband's. The surgeon stood next to her and whispered something; the woman nodded and her sobs subsided. Her shoulders relaxed and her breathing became more regular. The surgeon whispered again, pointing to the monitors and to the patient's chest and then gently putting his hand on the patient's arm. He was, I thought, explaining how life leaves the body—the last contractions of the heart, the irregular breaths, the final comfort of her presence. The woman nodded and began crying softly and stroking her husband's arm.

I wanted to join them but could not bring myself to do so. I pulled the curtains closed and went back to the nursing station to wait.

Thirty minutes passed before the surgeon stepped out. Soon after, the patient's wife appeared; her husband had died. She thanked us, smiled weakly, and walked out of the ICU.

She sent me a note a couple of weeks after her husband died. The stationery was cream-colored with slate-

blue borders, and her handwriting had long sweeping tails
that crisscrossed over the note. She wrote that although
her husband did not die at home, as she had always hoped,
he had died a dignified and peaceful death. "And that,"
she wrote, "was all we really wanted."

I kept that note with me for a long time afterward as a
reminder of what doctors could do. And long after I had
filed it away in my "Patient Correspondence" file, I would
reach into my white coat pockets as if the note were still
there and fall back on my memories of that morning as if
they could encourage me forward.

I stopped slipping away from my dying ICU patients
and their families. Instead with my hand in my pocket, I
would usher the families into the ICU. I would bring them
to their loved one's bedside and close the curtains around
not them but us. I would point to the irregularities on the
monitor and describe the characteristic last breaths of the
dying. I would touch family members, embrace those who
looked particularly lost, and tell them of the final comfort
of their presence.

I never discussed that morning's events or the contents of the woman's note with my former attending. I
never revealed how his deviation from the norm affected
me. I never told him that it was as if a shade had lifted ever
so slightly, letting in the first rays of light, and that from
that moment on, I would believe that I could do something
more than cure.

This narrative, then, is my acknowledgment to him.

Chapter 5 _____

M AND M _____

If you poke a hole from the belly into the diaphragm and, with your fingers, clear away the cobweblike tissues that separate the heart from the spine, there will be just enough space back there to fit your entire arm. And if you put a small incision along the base of the neck, as you do when you remove an esophagus, you might even see, if your forearm is long enough, the tips of your fingers poking out while your elbow remains enveloped by the soft, rubbery stomach and a flap of liver.

It's tempting to leave your arm in that warm, reassuring space. On the back of the forearm, you can feel the hardness of the vertebral bones, at the tips of the fingers, the coolness of open air, and at the elbow, the slithering contractions of the small bowel. But what you will marvel at most, and what will make you keep your arm there for just a few seconds longer than you probably should, is the sensation you notice against the patch of skin on the underside of your wrist, the most tender area where mothers gauge the temperature of milk for their babies.

Against that small swath of skin, and squirming of its own accord, you will feel the strong, twisting contractions of the heart. And it will remind you as you look down at the open belly and warm skin and bloodstained instruments on the table that the person whose body embraces you is very much alive.

Surgical residency is infamously difficult, so a month before I graduated from medical school, I polled my favorite surgery residents for advice.

"Sleep when you can, eat when you can," said one.

"Let your fingers do the walking," said another, pointing to the telephone.

"See a donut, eat a donut," said yet another.

One resident told me to draw up a list of the five most important things in my life and then cross out every one of them except the first. "That's all you'll have time for during internship," he said, "and maybe even not much of it at that."

I kept mental notes on these aphorisms, imagining myself passing them on to others one day. But of all the pithy observations, there was only one that I ever used.

Rob had completed his general surgery residency and was in his last year of subspecialty training when I worked with him. When not operating he displayed an array of nervous, tic-like movements that ranged from machine-gun-fire blinking to bouncing on his toes to passing his hands through his brown bristle-brush hair.

Despite the never-ending display of frenetic movements, Rob was the most even-keeled resident I had ever worked with. It helped, too, that he managed to find humor in situations that sent most residents screaming off the edge. He was supremely confident and gave me more responsibility and independence than I had ever experienced. I showed my medical student gratitude by throwing myself like a human shield into Rob's less savory scut. I made the calls to cranky radiology scheduling clerks, drew blood from ornery patients, and regularly ran interference with demanding attending surgeons. "Make sure to ask Dr. Miller a question about amputations," Rob would whisper to me before rounds. "He loves that stuff and it will keep him out of my hair for a while."

When I finally went to Rob for advice, I was hoping for the secret of sanity in residency training.

I caught Rob as he was wheeling a patient back to the ICU from the operating room. "Let me think about it a second," he said, grabbing his patient's chart and walking toward the nurses' station.

It was quiet in the ICU. All the patients appeared to be sleeping, and some of the nurses were away on their lunch break. The floor, freshly waxed, glistened under the fluorescent lights. Rob sat at the nurses' station writing his postoperative note. I saw his knee jiggling underneath the table and could not figure out how he kept his pen still enough to write.

Rob closed the chart and motioned for me to move closer to him. "All right, Pauline," he said. "Here's my advice." Not a single part of him was moving; I smiled, thinking that this sudden seriousness might be part of a playful game.

Rob looked straight at me. "Somewhere along the line," he said, "you are going to kill one of your patients."

I shook my head, not sure I had heard him correctly. I knew patients would die under my care, but my role was to save, not kill, them.

Rob leaned back in his chair, still looking at me. "You may not mean it, but it's going to happen." He sat there, absolutely still. I could hear the breathy chorus of ventilators in the background.

"Pauline," he finally said. "This happens to all of us. It's part of the job if you're in it for long enough. You'll just come to accept it as part of the learning process."

Rob stood up. He put his hand up to his head, removed his surgical cap, and began running his fingers through his hair. The nervous movements had started up again, and I saw him anxiously looking in the direction of the operating rooms.

"Listen," he said, now walking to the ICU exit. "When it happens to you, you call me and we'll talk. You'll understand then. Really."

As the doors closed behind him, I wondered if what he had said to me was really true. For days afterward all I could think about every time I saw one of my residents or attending surgeons was "Whom did you kill?" While I went about my duties as senior medical student and budding intern, I wanted to stop every one of them and ask about that patient. How did it happen? Did you know you were doing it? Or did you only realize it later after the fatal mistake?

Like some festering ulcer, Rob's words gnawed away at my gut. I remembered his promise to talk, but when it finally happened to me during my second year of residency, I never talked about it with him or with any of my residency colleagues or even with my family. Instead, all I could wonder then as I watched other surgeons walk by was "How do you ever get over it?"

In the early 1970s, Charles Bosk, then a sociology graduate student at the University of Chicago, spent eighteen months observing a surgical training program. At the time Bosk was interested in how surgeons as a professional group dealt with error. He rounded with them, attended conferences, and went to the operating room. He became, in essence, a full-fledged member of the surgical service.

During that year and a half, Bosk discovered a professional culture that demanded the highest level of competence among its members: infallibility in a highly variable world. He also noted that the surgeons' group identity was intimately linked to that drive for perfection. While surgeons were free to choose individually how they cared for patients, they had to be prepared throughout their training and careers to be entirely accountable to the professional group for any decisions they made.

Bosk observed that insofar as death was concerned, this accounting was done primarily in Morbidity and Mortality, or M and M, conferences. These conferences provided an opportunity for the surgeons of the hospital to learn by discussing recent surgical deaths and complications. According to Bosk, however, M and M was also a rite where a strong sense of professional coherence was instilled into an otherwise highly independent group of individuals. As Bosk phrases it, these conferences were a special ritual "for witnessing [these errors], resolving the confusion they create, and incorporating them into the group's history and the individual's biography." And this ritual function was so important that even "those accustomed to letting others cool their heels" cleared all other obligations in order to attend M and M.

Bosk's findings remain valid today. If you throw around the words "patient death" to a group of surgeons, they will almost reflexively want to go to M and M. And other than the patients discussed and the surgeons involved, there is little variation in the way M and M's are run across the country. Even the manner of presentation—always the passive voice and delivered as flatly as possible—is unchanged from Bosk's experiences. While there are some exchanges that seem calm and reasoned, others are impassioned, and the raised voices and emotions always point, however subconsciously, to something more than a difference of opinion among professional colleagues.

Occasionally deaths are chalked up to a disease's natural course. More often, surgeons identify a single mistake and categorize it as an error in technique, judgment, diagnosis, or management. Whatever the category, by the end of the conference, the surgeons in the room almost inevitably come to the same conclusion: the responsibility for the error—and thus the patient's death—lies squarely on the shoulders of the attending surgeon.

In rereading Bosk's work recently (my sister gave me the book when I was in medical school), I found the familiarity of his subjects to be disconcerting; it was as if Bosk had dipped into my brain and culled out memories of M and M. I heard the interrogations from the audience and saw the offending surgeon standing alone under the spotlight. My gut churned as the surgeon under fire shifted, wincing as the old wound was flayed open once again.

Having stood there in that line of fire, I know what that wound is. It has little to do with the conference or the attacks or even the error itself. Rather, it is that horrible sense that maybe it *was* your fault, that maybe you *are* truly to blame for your patient's death.

Harold "Dutch" Smulder was a sixty-five-year-old World War II veteran, reformed alcoholic, and unrepentant three-pack-a-day smoker who developed cancer of the esophagus when I was a second-year surgical resident. Unruly tufts of blond and white hair offset the downward drag of his jaw, and his long face had a softness to its contours, as if there were a prominent layer of fat stowed underneath his facial skin. He was the last branch of his family tree, a gruff, almost flinty lifelong bachelor who never gave people a lot to hang on to in conversation.

I, of course, fell for him almost immediately.

In the week before his operation, I visited him twice a day for formal work rounds and then would stop by his room during my nights on call. If I prodded, Dutch would warily spit out a few anecdotes about the war. If I laughed hard enough at one of his jokes, he would guffaw, his rubbery lips opening wide and his eyes disappearing in the depths of his cheeks like one of those Chinese wrinkled dogs.

I liked to think that Dutch enjoyed my visits and even developed a kind of teasing affection for me. One evening Dutch complained that he had had problems with the lunch. I immediately thought of his tumor, alarmed that it might be growing so quickly that we would not be able to remove it. He watched me for a moment and then began to laugh. "It's not because of the tumor, Doc," he said, patting me on the shoulder. "It's because the food in this joint is so damn awful."

The night before Dutch's operation, I went to his room with a consent form in hand. The attending surgeon, I told

Dutch, was famous for his skill, particularly with this procedure, and he would perform the surgery while the chief resident and I would assist. Given the scope of the operation, Dutch would likely be in the intensive care unit for a few days afterward.

Dutch nodded and looked at the form. He silently pointed to the list of potential complications that I had written at the bottom. Some of them, such as leaks from the new connections, were specific to this operation; others, like wound infections, were potential risks of any surgery. I rushed through my explanation; I did not want Dutch to be frightened. "There is a 30 percent risk of some kind of complication and maybe a 5 percent risk of death," I said.

Dutch looked at me. His mouth was twisted, and he fingered a loose thread on his hospital-issue gown. "So you think this operation is the right thing to do, Doc?" he asked.

I knew what I had read in books and medical journals, and Dutch fit the profile of the esophageal cancer patient with the best possible chances of benefiting from surgery. Of course, the operation would have to go smoothly, and he would have to recover, but those seemed like such minor steps to me.

Without hesitation, I looked at Dutch and nodded. "Yes, Dutch. The operation is the right thing to do."

Dutch smiled and then took the pen from me, writing his name in shaky script on the line reserved for patients.

"Carry on, Doc," he said. "Carry on."

I was on call the night after Dutch's operation. The operation had gone exceedingly well. Through an incision in his abdomen and one at the base of his neck, we had removed

Dutch's entire esophagus. Since the tumor appeared to be localized to a small segment of the esophagus, we had likely given Dutch the best chance possible of survival.

And I, the member of the surgical team with the slimmest limbs, had been the one who, with my entire arm in Dutch's chest, had confirmed that we could pull his stomach up and reconnect his gut once again.

At 2:00 a.m. on the night after the operation, I made a quick visit to the surgical ICU. The usual facility was under renovation, so Dutch and the other ICU patients were in a temporary unit, one originally designed for less critical patients. Dutch was in the corner room. He still had not awakened from surgery and had a tube to help him breathe. The nurses had placed his hands in soft restraints to prevent him, in a moment of confusion, from pulling on the tube or any of his extensive wiring.

"Dutch," I whispered to him. "It's Dr. Chen."

He squeezed my hand in hazy recognition and then fell back asleep.

I left the ICU but a half hour later received a frantic page to return. Because Dutch was in that corner room, no one had seen him wriggle his right arm out of the restraint and then, in his sedated state, pull out his breathing tube.

By the time I arrived, Dutch's heart rate had dropped from 95, when I last visited him, to 60. He looked bluish, and I felt the skin on my own inner wrists turn cold.

One nurse was struggling to compress Dutch's chest, while others had wheeled the code cart into the small room and were drawing up medications from vials. I could hear the hospital operator's airy voice—we called her Glinda because she sounded like the good witch from *The Wizard of Oz*—repeating over and over again on the hospital PA, "Code Blue, Surgical ICU. Code Blue, Surgical ICU." I scrambled to the head of the bed and asked the unit secretary to get hold of the senior resident, who was on call from home that night.

The respiratory therapist and I first tried to use a mask to give Dutch oxygen. Each of us pulled up on Dutch's jaw and cheeks, sealing his flesh against the plastic to prevent any oxygen from escaping around the mask. The swelling in his throat, however, obstructed his trachea, and each of our administered breaths of oxygen only blew up his cheeks and dislodged the mask from our hands. Looking over my shoulder, I could see that Dutch's heart rate had slowed further, to 45.

Dutch was suffocating.

I called out for a breathing tube and looked inside Dutch's mouth. All I could see were pink swollen tissues instead of the dark tunnel that should have been his airway. I tried to force the tube down Dutch's throat twice, unsuccessfully. After the second attempt I looked up at the cardiac monitor again and saw that Dutch's pulse had drifted down further, to 30. The nurses were giving atropine to try to reverse the slowing rhythms of his heart, but we all knew that without oxygen, everything else was futile.

There are moments in the hospital when time seems to suspend itself. Each second draws itself out, and actions take on a slow, dreamlike quality, as if they are replaying themselves even as they occur. As the events unfold before you, observer and participant, you find yourself reacting not with the rational and deliberate thoughts you have been taught, but as if nature, not some professor, had etched the responses into your neurons. In these moments when you are faced with life or death, it is as if the distillation of all those hours caring for sick patients bubbles to your brain's surface, and what you find yourself doing feels as natural as the most primal of reactions.

Looking at Dutch's falling heart rate and his swollen neck, I realized that he needed a cricothyroidotomy, an inch-long incision just below the Adam's apple for a breathing tube. I asked for Betadine, a scalpel, and a sterile surgical clamp. I had performed a cricothyroidotomy only once before—on a pig in an Advanced Cardiac Life Support course the week before internship—but my hands acted as if the routine had been embedded in my genes. I poured the Betadine over Dutch's neck, and the brown liquid splashed over the bed and onto my scrubs. I felt the flatness below his Adam's apple and drew the knife down. I pushed the blunt surgical clamp toward the back of his throat, plunging it into his airway and spreading the steel jaws to create a hole large enough for a breathing tube. I pushed the tube into Dutch's neck and down toward his dying lungs.

We beat against Dutch's chest, infused drugs, and delivered enough joules of electricity to his body to leave oval burn marks where our paddles had been placed. His lifeless body slid on the bed, pushed by our persistent, rhythmic chest compressions, and every time we delivered a shock from the defibrillator pads, his arms and legs would flail like the limbs of a rag doll that had been thrown across the room. The breathing tube was working; the level of oxygen in his blood was probably better than mine at that moment, but we were, ultimately, too late. His heart would never start up again.

Forty-five minutes later, I pronounced him dead.

Ten minutes after that the senior resident arrived. "Oh, shit," I heard him whisper as soon as he caught sight of Dutch's dead body. I followed him into Dutch's room, but he ignored me, picking through the scattered EKG tracings on the bed and the lab results strewn on the floor. "What the hell happened?" he asked, looking not at me but at Dutch's body. I told him, and he threw the scraps of paper he had collected back on the floor.

"Damn it, Pauline. You should have coded him longer, at least an hour. I don't care if his heart could not start up after forty-five minutes."

I felt my own drop to the floor.

"Now we are going to have to present this guy at M and M and give some reason for why he died." He walked over to one of the phones to call the attending. "Shit," he repeated over and over again.

He suddenly stopped and looked at me. "No, Pauline, I am not going to present this case," he said. "*You* are going to do it. You are doing the M and M."

I listened to him talk to the attending over the phone and then went to look at Dutch once more. The nurses were clearing away the needles and blood and preparing his body for the morgue. He looked cold and pale; the breathing tube sprouted up from where I had slit his neck.

I stood there without moving. I thought of the summer when I was six. I had gone down the pool steps to swim, my legs descending as if of their own accord. As the water of the pool came to my chin, I felt my right leg swing out and step down, pulling me into the shimmering whiteness of water. I saw the sunlight disappear along with my breath, swallowed up by the brightness. My feet touched the bottom, and I struggled to push up with my toes. As my head broke the surface, I began to scream, only to sink back down, blinded by the bubbles of my own breath and silenced by the water that filled my mouth and lungs.

As I wept by Dutch's room, I felt as if I had fallen in the pool once again, each gasp giving me less and less air until I could breathe no more. Except that this time I had taken Dutch Smulder along.

. . .

I spent the following week thinking about Dutch, going over in my mind again and again each minute of that ill-fated resuscitation and the ten minutes I had spent alone with him beforehand. I tried to remember the squeeze of his hands, the placement of his wrist restraints, the cricothyroidotomy. I even dreamed that I had loosened the restraints as I left him earlier that night, and the dream was so vivid that I no longer could remember the truth.

But what could I say, I kept thinking that Friday morning after his death, to the attending surgeons, residents, and students sitting in front of me? I had dreaded M and M, but could I bring myself to say that it was I, not the confused patient, who had let his hands go?

From the stage of the lecture hall, I began presenting. "H.S. was a sixty-five-year-old-male with a past medical history significant for alcohol and tobacco abuse who presented two weeks ago with adenocarcinoma of the esophagus." Would the attending surgeons discover, I wondered as my voice droned on in that passive haze, that my dream had been the truth, that I had killed Dutch Smulder?

"H.S. underwent a transhiatal esophagectomy, complicated only by excessive facial and neck swelling. He remained intubated and on the ventilator postoperatively." As I spoke, I hardly noticed the notes melting in my hand but instead felt Dutch's heart against my wrist. I saw his open belly in the operating room and felt his swollen hand squeeze mine in the ICU. I heard him laughing a few nights before the surgery, making fun of the hospital food yet again.

"At two-forty a.m., the patient self-extubated." I bit my lip, trying to keep my voice and face impassive.

"A code was called. An emergent cricothyroidotomy

was performed." The scene flashed in front of my eyes once again: the Betadine splashing over his throat, the knife against his neck, and the clamp entering his trachea. I saw Dutch's skin and lips become blue and heard the beeping from his heart monitor drift off.

"Despite forty-five minutes of resuscitative efforts, H.S. was pronounced dead at three-twenty-seven a.m." I emphasized the "forty-five minutes," sure that I would otherwise be held accountable. The room was silent and the audience stared at me grimly.

The interim chief of surgery at the hospital stepped up to the podium. I had searched for him the day after Dutch's death, recounting the events and hoping for absolution. "Well, that's tough," he replied. "Let's see what happens at M and M."

His eyes bore into me now, and I suddenly became aware of being alone, up front and center stage. "Doctor," he asked, "what is the standard of care for patients with esophageal cancer?"

I answered with all that I had read and researched, but with every successful answer came another more detailed and probing question. Questions from the audience rushed forth about every possible detail of Dutch's last day until all was quieted by the final question.

"So, Doctor," asked the department chief. "How do you account for this death?"

I heard the clock in the room ticking. I opened my mouth. The water rushed in once again.

The department chief stepped toward me and began to address the room. "I've talked to the nurses who were working that night, to the nurse in charge, and to all the doctors involved in H.S.'s case." He paused just long enough for me to cast one more glance at the impassive audience. "My frank feeling on this case," he continued, "is that this unfortunate death was due to an unacceptable temporary ICU setup. I've gone back and looked at that corner room, and even I cannot see how anyone could have adequately monitored a sedated, intubated, fresh post-operative patient."

I remember hearing a murmur of agreement through the audience. Another attending surgeon volunteered the story of her own patient who had been in that corner room and poorly monitored. After that, the department chief excused me to go back to my seat.

I had been officially absolved of guilt.

As the conference ended, a few attending surgeons and residents walked by and patted me on the back. The department chief put his hand on my shoulder. "Good job with that code," he said. "These things happen."

I walked out of the room, and that was it. Although that attending surgeon would never again perform an operation like Dutch's in that hospital, and a new ICU replaced the temporary one, clinical life continued as it always had. The senior resident smiled whenever we were on call together, the interim department chief grilled others at M and M, and no one ever mentioned Dutch's name again. And while I ached to share my grief with others besides my best friend, Celia, I could not help but also believe that there was nothing more to do and thus nothing more to say. Dutch Smulder was best left buried along with all the other initialed patients on that morning's handout in the annals of the department's Morbidity and Mortality conference.

There is something intensely personal about surgery. Our hands are in our patients' bodies, caressing them as no lover ever could. All the usual assumptions about propriety are cast away, and we literally hurl ourselves into the path of a disease. We use our fingers to break apart the filmy webs of infected loculations, our cupped palms to scoop out clotted blood, and our gloved fingernails to pry free adherent loops of bowel. Our work is an extension of ourselves, but we come to believe much more—that we *are* our work.

That lesson starts early in our training. I remember not so much the first patient nor the first incision I ever sewed closed, but the visit I made the following day. I was the junior medical student on the vascular surgery service, and that morning the head of the department joined rounds. Our large group entered the patient's room. After the attending asked the patient several questions and did a cursory physical exam, we all turned to leave. The attending surgeon suddenly spun around at the doorway and went back to pull down a part of the patient's incision dressing.

"Didn't you close this up?" he asked me.

I nodded, and he motioned for me to come to the patient's side. The closure looked beautiful to me; the edges were aligned perfectly, each stitch was evenly placed. Even the patient, despite having been pawed and gawked over, was beaming.

"Come over and admire your handiwork!" ordered the surgeon with a laugh. "It's pretty good, isn't it?" He chuckled. He wiggled his own delicate fingers in the air, as if to emphasize his point: our hands are our instruments, our interventions a direct extension of ourselves.

Over time, the line between our selves and our work blurs. We see a patient walking around and will identify that person as "I did her colon" or "I did his liver," as if we are responsible for that patient's actual part. These are narcissistic moments but ones that patients indulge in as well. More than once I have overheard my patients say, "That's Dr. Chen's work," while pointing to the scars I have left behind.

It is hardly surprising, then, that death for surgeons is more than a passive process. It is immensely and profoundly personal; it is about us. Surgeons will, for example, do everything possible to prevent a patient from dying "on the table." While trying to keep a patient alive in the OR is an honorable quest, I was struck as an intern by the ritual that occurred once death became inevitable. The attending surgeons would hastily do everything possible to close up and rush the patient out of the OR, even if that patient expired only a few minutes later in the ICU. The first time I saw this happen as an intern, these quick exits seemed superstitious. Later, after I witnessed the second such death, I asked my friend Celia why there had to be all this rushing about. "Because," she replied, having posed the same question a few days earlier to a chief resident, "a death in the OR means it was the surgeon's fault, and you have to do *everything* to prevent *that*."

Our fingers, no matter how nimble and graceful, are always tangled up with the fate of our patients, and when one of those patients dies, it is impossible to divest ourselves of that sense of responsibility. We torment ourselves with the what-ifs. Perhaps, if we had put that stitch in just a little differently or removed that cancer a little higher up or worked a little longer, then maybe our patient's course might have been different.

M and M, our professional ritual centered on death, attempts to heal the rents in our professional fabric caused by patient deaths. There are few other opportunities for surgeons to discuss death. We may mention it in passing, but we steadfastly reserve discussion for the conference, which will give us, as a group, ritual absolution. M and M requires a public accounting of loss and, in so doing, reconstructs the death into an event that affirms a core value of our professional identity: the need to be infallible in a highly variable world. In this way, M and M is like death rituals in other cultures; it seeks to transform death's loss into an affirmative experience.

Unfortunately, the very rituals that were meant to heal a community in death can also hinder that process. Peter Metcalf and Richard Huntington, two anthropologists who have studied rituals in funerary practices, write, "Whatever mental adjustments the individual needs to make in the face of death he or she must accomplish as best he or she can through or around such rituals as society provides. No doubt rites frequently aid adjustment. But we have no reason to believe that they do not obstruct it with equal frequency." In the case of M and M, death is viewed wholly through the lens of personal responsibility. Death is rendered optional, and mortality becomes a quantifiable and correctable error.

By defining death only as the result of errors, we erase the face of our patients and insert our own fiercely optimistic version of immortality. While admirable in some respects, this paradigm also denies our essential humanness. When we refuse to accept our own fallibility, we deny ourselves grief. In the end, then, M and M may prevent us from reaching what we so desperately want to achieve: the very best care for our patients.

There is a paradox to rituals. While they safeguard the status quo and control unpredictable individual variations, rituals can also inspire creativity. They can supply the framework needed to introduce new meaning to an event.

M and M has in recent years become the focus of a

new approach to death and dying. Long regarded as an instrument for denying death, M and M has more recently been transformed into one of the primary venues for incorporating end-of-life care initiatives and formally addressing the personal significance of patient deaths. In 2002 the American College of Surgeons issued a new mandate to improve end-of-life care training for surgeons. One of the key vehicles for this change has been the M and M conference. Internal medicine training programs have not only incorporated M and M into their training programs but have also begun to use this conference similarly as an educational tool for end-of-life care.

Perhaps the very characteristics that compel us to find fault first with ourselves—that profoundly personal stake in a patient's death—have transformed this ritual into something greater.

It has been twelve years since Dutch died. Although the attending surgeons at M and M chalked Dutch's death up to a problem in the temporary ICU's setup, I continued to ask myself for years about the course of events that night. What if I had taken extra care to tighten his wrist restraints the first time I saw him? What if I had resuscitated him for fifteen minutes more? What if I had not encouraged him to sign the operative consent?

I have cared for hundreds more patients since Dutch died, and with that experience, I understand the events of that night a little differently now, perhaps more like the interim department chief than the young resident I was. I have found some peace, but Dutch still comes back to me. He is a ghostly apparition who appears whenever I see a patient with esophageal cancer, perform a cricothyroidotomy, or run an emergency resuscitation.

And there is one other event that brings Dutch back. Each July 1, a new class of interns appears on the wards. I watch those interns, remember my first weeks, and then imagine what the years ahead hold for them. I wonder if they, too, will carry the same burdens as the rest of us.

That is when I see Dutch again, signing his name for me and telling me to carry on.

A year after I had finished all my training, a patient died on the wards of the liver surgery service. An intern had examined the patient, left the room, and within minutes was called back when a nurse noticed that the patient had become unresponsive. A team that included the covering attending surgeon tried to resuscitate the patient for close to an hour without success.

One of the nurses called me that afternoon. "I know you are not covering, but would you mind going to see that intern?" she asked.

I walked over to the floor. It looked no different than usual. Nurses were busy in patient rooms, phlebotomists walked by carrying their plastic picnic baskets filled with gleaming empty tubes and requisition slips fluttering. I walked into the small office reserved for interns. Papers and films were piled about haphazardly. The intern sat huddled over a computer.

I introduced myself. For a moment I saw fear flicker over his eyes, as if he expected me to bawl him out.

Instead, I asked him what had happened and how he felt. He was cagey at first. Then I told him about Dutch. I told him how hard it was for me and how, years later, I still thought about Dutch. "But you know what?" I said to the intern. "I think I am a better and more compassionate surgeon because of Dutch."

He sat there, face impassive. I was not sure if I had said too much.

But a couple of days later, there was a knock at my door. My office was set off a corridor in another wing of the hospital, nestled among cardiologists and far from other liver surgeons. Visitors were rare.

I opened the door and it was the intern. His face was still impassive.

"Just wanted to say thank you," he mumbled.

As he quickly turned to walk away, I only had time to say, "No problem." But I spent the rest of the day with Dutch's grinning face in the back of my mind.

Chapter 6

THE VISIBLE WOMAN

For much of my childhood, I was convinced that behind the smiling blue eyes of my pediatrician, Dr. Kirkland, lurked an omniscient being. He discerned not only insidious diseases but also the candy I had snitched from my mother's do-not-touch shelf, the dirt I had swallowed on a schoolyard challenge, and the litany of lies I used whenever I was late for dinner.

I stewed for days about my annual visit, and in pre-exam penance, I adhered to a strict no-candy, no-nonsense regimen, believing that would wipe clear a year's worth of errant behavior. When I finally submitted on Dr. Kirkland's examining table to his looks into my eyes and ears, his gentle feel of my belly, and his rubber hammer's dead-on tap to my knees, I hardly let out a peep. There was too great a risk that he might discover my year's slips and report to my parents. He asked me about my teachers, about my friends, and about what I wanted to be when I grew up. When my mother piped up, filling in my skeletal replies, Dr. Kirkland would turn toward me, his back to my mother, and then repeat my mother's answers with his left eyebrow raised and a crooked grin on his face. I wondered if he knew the truth.

In the fifth grade, everything changed. I believed that I had discovered the key to Dr. Kirkland's omniscience. And I found it on the shelf of a local toy store that was going out of business.

Not much bigger than a Barbie doll, the Visible Woman was a do-it-yourself model kit, complete with unpainted plastic organs that you snapped inside a clear plastic female body. The box bore a mesmerizing repro-duction of the treasure within: white bones, blue lungs, red heart, and a plum-colored liver glistening beneath a glossy female shell, and lightning bolts of red and blue vessels streaking across transparent arms and legs. In the store I gingerly shook the box and angled it up to the light, hoping to turn the two-dimensional picture into three. I felt my heart pounding—I was holding the answer to Dr. Kirkland's powers.

For months afterward, I wheedled my parents about the Visible Woman, pulling out every psychological stop. With the Visible Woman I could learn anatomy, I told them. I could do a dissection without doing a real dissec-tion, I reasoned. And when those arguments appeared to have lost their force, I pulled out my biggest gun, one that I knew would be fail-proof with my immigrant parents: I could get a head start on medical school.

I was the kind of kid who made Halloween candy last until spring, so when the Visible Woman finally arrived at Christmas, I spent the first couple of days simply gazing at the picture on the box and relishing all that it promised. Then I spent a few weeks admiring all the parts. I lovingly fingered the plastic organs still attached to their stems, allowing my fingertips to memorize the slopes and grooves of each piece. I set the empty female shell up on my desk as a daily reminder of what was to come. I even started a notebook of anatomy, drawing the parts with colored pencils and then describing the function of each underneath. It was such sweet labor, drawn out to savor every bit of pleasure.

In the end, though, I never came close to putting my Visible Woman together. My younger brother and sister, now both doctors themselves but back then envious of the attention I paid to the Visible Woman, pulled most of the organs off their plastic vines and scattered them around the house and yard. My paint job on the remaining few dripped; the reds and blues blended to make everything purple. The clear casing fell off my desk and broke. Nevertheless, the Visible Woman's image lingered in my mind long after the bones, organs, and shell were gone. How could I forget the perfection of all those parts nestled within?

From that point on until my last pediatrician visit the year I left for college, I never saw Dr. Kirkland in the same way. While he continued to ask me questions—how I was doing in school, where I wanted to go to college, and even the potentially incriminating if I had a "special friend" yet—he no longer loomed quite as large. Instead, as he dimmed the room lights and peered into his lighted ophthalmoscope, I could look straight back, my eyes unblinking. I could stare beyond his black-rimmed glasses and squinting blue eyes and see not a reflection of myself but glossy see-through casing. A tangle of red blood vessels would appear against the backdrop of whiteness—a reflection of my eyeball through his lenses. And I would, for one moment, believe that I had seen the world as Dr. Kirkland did.

Doctors—like writers, artists, and spies—are professional people-watchers. More specifically, a doctor's work relies on the ability to discern, among thousands of biological cues, the underlying pathology. It is a skill that is part art, part science; and the more we can see, and sense, and sort, the better our care.

The "art" part requires a kind of clairvoyance, a sixth sense of how the pieces fit. It is, I believe, a true gift. There is something nearly miraculous when, among dozens of doctors who have been scratching their heads for days, one of those gifted souls will enter a patient's room and within minutes correctly make the diagnosis.

On the other hand, nearly everyone can learn the "science" part. The "science" is the ability to pick out the pieces while not necessarily knowing their relevance. Doctors begin learning that skill early on, starting with the cadaver and, later, fine-tuning it in the living. We learn to use our senses to discriminate among subtle variations— a certain vascular marking on the face, a splaying of the fingertips, and a sweet, almost candied breath. We dismantle people as art experts deconstruct paintings. Instead of seeing families gathered by the lake of a park or the stars in the sky, we see the purple and pink dots, the gray shading, and the yellow highlights.

Eventually we apply these skills not just to diagnosing but also to interpreting everything in our clinical world.

Deconstruction becomes our professional tool of understanding, and we rely on it to absorb increasingly complicated clinical problems. A patient in multisystem organ failure, when reduced to bodily systems—neurologic, pulmonary, cardiac, and so on—becomes manageable for even the most junior of residents. The wounds inflicted by the unpredictable ricocheting bullet become a distinct, potentially reparable set of injuries when the patient's abdomen is explored quadrant by quadrant. Even a liver transplant can be broken down into small, easily accomplished steps. By knowing all those pieces we give ourselves a sense of control over even the most daunting situations; and by practicing this skill over and over again, we get to be pretty good at it.

In the course of my training, I actually came to enjoy this deconstructing. It was mentally satisfying, like taking a box of jumbled puzzle pieces, organizing them, then arranging them into a perfect picture. The only problem was that I could not *stop* doing it. I did it almost constantly at work and then would find myself still doing it during my time off. I saw people in the grocery store or at restaurants, and my eyes would fixate on the loping gait, the barrel chest, or the finely wrinkled skin. *Stroke, emphysema, big-time smoker,* I would think. It was strangely thrilling, the way having X-ray vision might be.

Then one day my Aunt Grace, my mother's younger sister, asked me for some medical advice. Her surgeons had just created a hemodialysis graft using a small stretch of tubing to connect a vein to an artery in her upper arm. Her forearm blood vessels were tiny, and the graft there had collapsed over and over again, unable to support the high flow rates required by dialysis. When it finally clotted off, the surgeons went to her upper arm, hoping these marginally bigger vessels would be hardier.

That afternoon in her living room my aunt rolled up her sleeve to show me the new graft site. She had been shrinking over the last decade and now barely reached my chest. On her upper arm I saw the snakelike graft bulging beneath her skin, and a four-inch-long scar peppered with black nylon sutures. Her skin was red and, touching it, I felt only the pulse of my own fingers.

My mind began wandering. I saw the reddened incision open up, exposing a minuscule artery and vein. There was a swarm of blue sutures, each finer than hair, connecting the vessels to a graft. But the graft was not quivering with fresh, whooshing blood; it was purple with blood pooled solid.

I glanced over at her right arm, but it appeared as diminutive as the other. I looked down at my aunt's thighs, but when that skin evaporated away in my mind, those vessels, too, were hopelessly small. My mind raced ahead, skipping a year, maybe two. I saw each attempt by her surgeon, every new graft, clot off until my aunt had no lifeline at all.

I felt a pressure rising in my head, the same pressure that came every time I was left with pieces that could never come together. I had no answers, only a glimpse of her future. And from that moment on I could dwell on nothing else but.

When I was growing up, Aunt Grace liked to tell me why I would make a good doctor. "You're so good at listening to people," she said. "Patients are going to fill up your waiting room." Now, though, I could not bear to listen. With all my willpower, I tried to concentrate on her chatter while averting my eyes from her latest graft site and from the oxygen prongs in her nose. When she asked me a medical question, I held my breath, afraid that if I let go, my tenuous composure might falter.

For the next year and a half, whenever I left her—on the phone, at her house, or at the hospital—I would feel that pressure rising again in my head. The first few times, the pressure was throbbing, like a headache about to blossom. Later the pressure would appear only momentarily, as a prelude to a much more intense wave of grief.

The skill that had once simplified my life now left me very much alone, and the profession that had once promised the power of cure now made me utterly helpless.

She had been a part of my life from the beginning. Aunt Grace arrived in Cambridge a week before my birth, and although she ostensibly came over for graduate work, her real job during that first year in the United States was to help my mother manage a new marriage, a foreign country, her own graduate studies, and what would be a very colicky baby.

Aunt Grace had just graduated from Taiwan's top university and was an accomplished amateur athlete. In one of the photos from around that time, she is standing next to my mother and has the broad smile and easy stance of a woman whose body has become a second-nature instrument of grace. Her face is gorgeously full, like the fleshy pumpkins of New England Octobers, and her calves are round and strong. Thinking back now with the perspective of middle age, I cannot imagine how she managed in an apartment crowded with her sister, brother-in-law, inconsolable niece, and the memories of glory in a country half a world away.

But as a young child I had no concerns about my aunt's happiness nor about her past achievements. Instead, I thought only about my own hedonistic pursuits, and from an early age, those were centered on food. It was in this secret chase after adrenaline-rushing, mouth-tingling, mind-expanding tasty delights that my aunt and I formed our earliest bonds, a kind of gustatory collusion. She became the aunt who not only gave me the foods my mother would never let me eat, but also relished their sinfulness as much as I. From my Aunt Grace, I learned to drop teaspoonfuls of sugar into warm milk, sprinkle the same snowy crystals over rice, and eat Cap'n Crunch cereal straight out of the box. Wherever she was, she created a glucose heaven; and if I cautiously parroted my mother's admonitions, she would wave her hand, guffaw, and encourage me to have more while my mother was not around.

Although we saw her infrequently after she moved away, her stature continued to grow in my eyes. One of her first jobs was teaching. In my mind, she was no longer just my Aunt Grace but now also the teacher of students who were four or five years older than I. In her apartment beyond the paradisiacal kitchen, she had drawers filled with art supplies, workbooks, and projects from her classroom. It was my opportunity, however indirectly, to rub elbows with the big kids, and Aunt Grace turned it into a grand event. She would pull out the crayons and papers and workbooks, regale me with stories about her students, and then coo so sincerely over my art that I became utterly convinced of my ability to bypass kindergarten and go directly to the third grade. By the time she had her own children a few years later, I was busy with homework, my friends, and after-school activities, but I always felt a little envious of Aunt Grace's brood.

I saw my Aunt Grace less and less after college but spoke to her about half a dozen times during my residency. Her kidneys were failing, and I was learning about transplantation. A few years ago, I moved a couple of towns away from her. I was now a fully trained transplant surgeon, and she had been on the kidney transplant waiting list for seven years. On the rare occasions that she felt well we met for lunch.

My twin toddler daughters loved those visits with her as much as I had at their age; she and her family had now become their most reliable source of toys, potato chips, and Eskimo Pies. Over the course of each meal together, my aunt chewed on a few ice cubes, savoring the precious cool liquid of each but afraid that one cube too many would leave her breathless until she got dialyzed again. My daughters from their high chairs tossed over pieces of their lunch: clumps of rice, half-eaten baby corn, and mangled pieces of shrimp; and each time I leaned over to pick up their mess, I caught glimpse of my Aunt Grace's legs peeking out from under her pants, the once glorious calves shriveled and scarcely bigger, it seemed, than the bamboo chopsticks the twins were learning to use.

But after that second hemodialysis graft operation, there were no more lunches. The upper arm graft soon clotted, and her surgeons quickly made plans to put another in her left thigh.

"Will it stay open?" she asked me one day. "And what happens when there are no more arteries or veins left to graft?"

I held my breath for a moment and then began telling her. My fears about her future came spilling out and I could barely keep from crying. "And then an emergency transplant may be the only option," I finally told her. Given her tiny frame and the difficulties of finding a suitably sized kidney, I knew that would be nearly impossible.

She sat back and nodded. Her face was impassive, as if she had known all along. She paused for a few minutes—long enough for me to hear my own uneven breaths—and then said to me, "You know, Pauline, I used to be scared of the idea of a transplant. But I have such a great kidney doctor and heart doctor now. And you should see the people that come back to visit the dialysis center after they get a kidney. They look so good. They can eat anything they want, they can drink anything they want, and they say they have never felt better." She stopped, looked up at me, and waited for my response.

"We'll get you strong," I said.

My Aunt Grace grinned and then walked over to her kitchen. My daughters had been quietly shoveling down fistfuls of blueberries that my aunt had set out to keep them occupied while I examined her. They looked up as she approached, their eyes wide with delight and their cheeks and hands stained purple.

I ran to grab a napkin, but my aunt waved me away. She leaned over to the girls, her body, it seemed, only slightly bigger than theirs, and whispered, "So who would like an ice cream sandwich?"

In every doctor's life, there are patients who change forever the way you approach your work. We call these patients "index cases," but we rarely discuss them with one another, except as another "interesting" case. To do otherwise would be to admit a potentially embarrassing vulnerability.

In 1992, as part of a lecture later published in the *Annals of Internal Medicine*, a cardiologist named Hacib Aoun described one such case from his internship. The patient, Mr. D, had a rapidly progressing neurologic illness that "had turned him into an emaciated, wheelchair-bound, helpless soul." He represented the worst kind of patient for an intern: not only did Mr. D have a terminal disease, but he also suffered from multiple complications that demanded the ongoing attention of his intern, Dr. Aoun. One day the patient's girlfriend gave Dr. Aoun one of Mr. D's wildlife paintings and then later showed him a picture, taken three months earlier, of the patient posing in front of his paintings. The Mr. D in the picture bore no resemblance to the patient Dr. Aoun knew. As Aoun recalled:

> It hit me violently that I had lost sight of my patients as human beings and had begun to see them as a different species: the patient species. . . . The process of becoming a doctor is so protracted and arduous that it is easy to forget along the way the initial reasons and ideals for wanting to become a doctor, especially because the current medical curriculum is disease-oriented, not patient-oriented.

The circumstances of Hacib Aoun's own life make his comments more poignant than usual. Nine years before he delivered his lecture, a blood-filled tube had fractured in Aoun's fingers. The blood was from a teenager with leukemia who had been transfused multiple times. In 1986, three years after that accident, Aoun felt ill enough to seek medical help. Of that moment he wrote, "The mystery was solved, and the nightmare began." He was diagnosed with HIV.

Nonetheless, for the next five years Aoun spoke at medical schools and conferences, bringing attention to the issue of occupational injuries among physicians. As time went on, he became a passionate speaker on the quality of care for the terminally ill. And on the day after his talk was published, Hacib Aoun passed away.

I do not have a terminal illness; nor do I have the kind of equanimity that Dr. Aoun possessed. I do, however, struggle to reconcile what medicine has taught me so well with the very reasons that drew me to it in the first place. I want to cry for those in whose bellies I find disseminated tumors, but cannot for fear of being unable to see clearly enough to sew them closed. I want to sit and linger with my patients, but know that such inefficiency would never work in the clinical world. I want to be able to soothe my patients' suffering without the burden of knowing the inexorable future course of their diseases.

I have read Hacib Aoun's speech a dozen times. He and I are separated by nearly a generation of medical discoveries—Aoun might have had a very different prognosis had he been diagnosed with HIV today—but his words resonate with me as few others have. As he wrote, "We need to devote more time and attention to teaching attitudes, skills, and behaviors at the expense of the present preoccupation and fascination with technical knowledge."

Each time I read those words, Hacib Aoun reaches out to me beyond time. With dignity and unflinching candor, he tells me how I, with my own distinct future, might do it differently.

Around the time I started medical school, Harvard began an experiment in medical education. Based on an integrated approach to learning, Harvard's New Pathway program represented a radical departure from the century-old reductionist paradigm.

Until the early twentieth century, physicians learned through apprenticeships or in medical schools where standards varied tremendously. In 1910 the Carnegie Foundation commissioned educator Abraham Flexner to study the status of American medical schools. The recommendations from the resulting work, often referred to as the Flexner Report, were the impetus for a series of sweeping reforms in medical education. Medical schools began standardizing their curriculum and teaching clinical work in the context of a basic science foundation. The Flexner Report influenced over a century of American medicine and was in many ways responsible for transforming a once uneven health care system into one of the best in the world.

One of the points that Flexner took care to explicate is the proper order of courses in medical school, with four years to include two years of basic science work followed by two years of clinical learning. The first two years are further broken down into the fundamental science blocks, the first year being devoted to learning normal human anatomy and physiology and the second year focusing on abnormal physiology and the disruptions of disease.

I began medical school over seventy-five years after Flexner published his report, but my school's curriculum still followed Flexner's guidelines nearly perfectly. As talented as some of my teachers were, I spent most of my first year and much of my second wondering about the relevance of all the names, formulas, and pathways I was committing to memory. A few times during those first two years, the professors would mention in passing how a particular fact might be important for patient care. I remember carefully writing down these isolated nuggets of information, encircling them with stars and exclamation points.

Most of the coursework felt like mental drudgery, and when I asked my classmates about their feelings, they chuckled in empathy. Mary, the preternaturally calm lab partner, finally said, "Pauline, it's like learning to read. Just think of these years as memorizing the words."

Harvard's New Pathway curriculum, however, did not divide the sciences; instead, it was grounded in problem-based learning and included "lectures, labs, weekly structured learning experiences focused on humanistic aspects of medicine, and clinical experiences designed to foster humanism and the doctor-patient relationship." Single cases were the lens with which to view all the pieces; the New Pathway students learned the disciplines as a cohesive and coordinated whole, as part of a larger picture. Proponents of this revolutionary change believed that this approach to medical education would result in more integrated, and therefore more humanistic, patient care.

A little over a decade later, educators looked at the impact of the New Pathway program on its students. The experiment had, it seemed, worked. They found that the first set of students to have gone through the curriculum felt more prepared to practice humanistic medicine than their traditionally educated counterparts and had more confidence in dealing with patients with psychosocial problems. Since 1985 other medical schools have attempted to start programs similar to the New Pathway program, overhauling segments of their curriculum in order to offer more integrated education to young doctors-to-be.

This new approach to medical education may be one of the answers to improving our future, for it emphasizes above all the importance of relationships—between science and art, between mind and body, between individuals. It is that sense of shared humanity, rather than the deconstruction of it, that may ultimately be the most powerful antidote to human suffering. And it may be the key to how doctors can do better.

At the end of his talk, Aoun wrote of the search for "that good physician who would say, 'I understand that this illness is happening to *you,* but *we* will face it together.' " He went on:

> Because it is particularly in cases of catastrophic or incurable illnesses that the role of the physician is more, not less, important, let me suggest that the fewer the therapeutic options available, the greater your involvement with the patient should be. When there is no cure, there is still much to be done to alleviate suffering.

My Aunt Grace had believed in my ability to listen to people. She knew about the experience of illness and understood how listening to patients—*being* with them—could transform suffering. In her niece, she saw someone who might be able to do that.

But over the years of training, I had forgotten that part of doctoring. I had learned to embrace the deconstruction of my work while ignoring the connections between the pieces. I had neglected the humanity I shared with patients and nearly trivialized its bearing on illness. I had focused on the Visible People and then forgotten Dr. Kirkland's familiar questions about friends, family, and "special others." While I might have believed at one time that I would practice a new, more humane kind of medicine, those hopes had somehow along the way vanished.

But not for my Aunt Grace. She would not let me forget. The woman who had helped me first find joy would also be the one who would show me what I had lost.

One afternoon about a year ago my aunt called me. I had sent her a draft of an article I was writing on brain death and organ donation. I thought her story would add an interesting personal perspective, but I wanted her consent.

My aunt had just returned home from a three-month hospitalization, much of it in an ICU. Her voice on the phone was barely audible; each sentence seemed to exhaust her.

"I think it's wonderful, Pauline," she said. "I'm excited because I think other people can learn from my experience." I could hardly bear to hear her struggle, so although I was thrilled with her encouragement, I suggested to her that we talk more another time.

"Yes, let's do that," she replied. "But I want you to do one thing for me."

I waited for her to continue. My aunt had always been intensely private, so I was guessing that she would want me to conceal her identity. I tried to fill in the words for her, so as not to have her expend any more energy. "Don't worry, Auntie," I said. "I will change your identity enough so that no one will know it's you."

I heard her raspy breath on the other end of the line. "It's not that, Pauline," she said. "You do what you wish there." There was another long pause as she struggled to catch her breath. "I only want one thing. I want you to emphasize your uncle and your cousin." For the first time, pulled away from my preoccupation with her grafts and vessels and transplant candidacy, I thought of my uncle and cousin. I thought of their lives for the last decade, marked by the overwhelming care for my aunt.

"They have been here for me always; they have listened to me always. Your uncle has taken such good care of me, and your cousin has helped him. They have sacrificed so much." Her voice began to falter; I could hear her forcing the last words out. "I owe everything to them. These two have been far more important than anything I have experienced or I can say. My story is also about them."

Three weeks later, my aunt died.

I was with her that morning; and as I had seen before in others, her breathing was labored, the air gurgling as it passed through her throat. At first she seemed delirious, swatting at an unyielding itch between her shoulder blades. My cousin had spent the night with her, scratching her itch, readjusting her oxygen mask, massaging her legs. When my uncle arrived in her room, a gentle wave of tranquillity passed over my aunt, from her face to her toes. Her furrowed brow began to relax and her drawn-up knees slowly fell flat.

I left my uncle and cousin, and less than an hour later, they called to tell me that my aunt had finally passed away. She had become progressively more peaceful, and in the end they sat there, simply being with her, as they had always done.

III

REAPPRAISAL

Chapter 7

FIRST, DO NO HARM

The barber was the first to notice them. He was washing Sam's hair, as he had for the last twenty years, when he felt those two marble-sized rocks trapped under the skin.

"Did you hit your head recently?" he asked his client.

Sam sat up, his head covered with suds. He lifted his arm out from beneath the black plasticized apron to feel where the barber's fingers had stopped.

"I've got to call Joanne," he said.

Sam had had a liver transplant two years earlier for hepatitis C and liver cancer, and since that time, he depended on his wife, Joanne, to oversee the slew of routine clinic visits, to organize his fistfuls of pills, and to maintain the rigorous schedule of follow-up CAT scans that would detect metastases. Sam, who had started up one of the most successful investment firms in Los Angeles, was more than capable of doing all this himself, but it was Joanne who had the remarkable knack of caring for others.

Their partnership began on a blind date in the 1950s. Joanne was a single mother and recently divorced. "I was shunned back then," Joanne told me once during one of Sam's clinic visits. "But Sam drove up with a beautiful car and opened the door of his car for me. I thought he was the perfect gentleman." After their marriage Sam adopted Joanne's son and had two more children with her. "Sam told me that the only thing I was responsible for was raising the children. He would take care of the rest. But he always knew that I had the harder job—trying to bring up three children to be happy and loving adults. Sam used to say that if our kids accomplished half of what I wanted for them, they would end up being president of the United States."

In recent years Joanne had devoted herself to her husband's complicated medical care. And Sam believed, as did I, that she was the primary reason for his remarkable clinical course. In the two years since the transplant Sam had returned only twice to the hospital, once for appendicitis and once for an episode of mild rejection.

That afternoon Joanne called us. Her voice was shaking. She, too, had felt the ominous, hard irregularity of those bumps when Sam returned home from the barbershop. A week later the pathology report from our biopsies confirmed Sam's and Joanne's worst fears: the cancer had spread.

Sam started chemotherapy but a third scalp mass soon appeared. Two weeks later Joanne called us again. Sam was acting slightly confused, and an MRI scan of his head revealed a new metastasis in his brain. Given the rapid progression of his cancer, our guess was that this new tumor would grow and, in as little as a couple of weeks, Sam would suffer from seizures and even become comatose. We told Joanne and Sam that their only option at this point would be to irradiate the brain metastasis; the radiation would impede but not cure Sam's cancer.

A couple of days later Joanne called my office. I recognized her soft, warbling voice on the other end of the line. Sam was with the physical therapist at the moment, so she had sneaked off to another part of the house to call me.

"How is he?" I asked.

"He seems all right. But I'm so anxious about these brain things," she said with a sigh. I imagined her huddled over a phone in a corner, whispering into the receiver. "Every time he forgets something, I'm afraid it's grown. Then I realize that we both tend to forget things all the time, that this is nothing new." Joanne asked me again about the radiation. She and Sam had wanted to spend a few days thinking it over before going ahead with any treatment. How much time would Sam have with it and how much without it, she wanted to know. What would be the side effects? Would he still get chemotherapy? Suddenly, I heard her sobbing on the other end of the line.

"When do you know," she asked when she finally caught her breath, "when you have done enough?"

I stared up at the white ceiling of my office, trying to imagine what Joanne was feeling at that moment. I knew she wanted someone who could both empathize and help her decide. I rifled through my mental files for an answer that might clarify everything. What had I read about metastatic liver cancer and radiation and survival? I searched for the answers that would allow me to say with quiet confidence "No, Sam should not choose the radiation" or "Yes, it would make sense for Sam's brain to be irradiated." But there was not even a distant memory of some study or trial or article that might help.

Finally, still struggling with that memory void, I told Joanne the truth. And the truth was that I really did not know.

Hanging in Room 15 among the other paintings and sculptures that make up the Victorian Spectacle collection of London's Tate Britain museum is a painting so well etched in my memory that I no longer remember the first time I saw it. The painting depicts daybreak in a small country cottage. A corner lamp highlights two figures: a young patient on the verge of recovery, with pink rising in her cheeks, and a serious physician whose intense paternal gaze seems to hold the answers to his patient's mortal struggle.

The Doctor, first exhibited in 1891, was the work of Luke Fildes, a Victorian painter well known for his powerful images of social injustice and poverty. Fildes drew from his own memories in painting *The Doctor;* his eldest son had died on Christmas morning 1877. Despite his son's death, the artist remained grateful to the physician, Dr. Gustavus Murray, and *The Doctor* not only paid homage to Dr. Murray but was also an attempt "to put on record the status of the doctor in our own time."

That status had changed dramatically. Fildes and his contemporaries had been witness to a succession of medical discoveries that resulted in enormous changes in the public's general welfare. Physicians and surgeons standardized their training and methods, abandoned antiquated notions like bloodletting and intestinal purgatives, and incorporated anesthesia and sterile techniques into their practices. The body was no longer a mysterious repository of disease but a rational, potentially reparable biological machine.

And doctors were the human purveyors of the revolution. Their ability to treat diseases empowered physicians, and that empowerment soon translated into an urge to treat not selectively but almost indiscriminately. The implicit meaning of the converse—doing nothing at all—came to represent a willful refusal of power and strength over disease.

That we can fend off disease and death through our actions is an intoxicating notion. I should know; it fueled many of my sleepless nights through training. There is no mistaking the heady exhilaration you feel when you walk into the cool and ordered operating room, pull out all the technical gadgetry and wizardry of the moment, and within a few hours solve the essential problem. Surgery is a specialty defined by action. As a student of mine once said, "Surgeons *do* something about a problem, not just sit around and think about it."

But surgeons are not alone in this doer's paradise. While surgery, particularly liver transplantation, represents an extreme, even physicians in specialties with little or no "invasive" procedures feel compelled to *do*. A patient visits with a problem, and the appointment is incomplete without a prescription for medications or tests or some tangible diagnosis.

Even medicine's essential framework for approaching clinical problems—the treatment algorithm—presumes physician action. Frequently diagrammed in textbooks and medical journals, these algorithms outline step-by-step therapeutic plans for different diseases. For every point along the algorithm there are several possible outcomes that in turn may have several of their own possible therapeutic options. On no branch of the decision tree, however, is there a box reserved for *Do nothing* or *Hold tight* or *Sit on your hands.* Instead, if no treatment is required, we describe the waiting as an active, not a passive, period. *Treat with intravenous antibiotics for six weeks and then reassess* may be part of the algorithm. Or we may decide on a course of what is euphemistically termed *expectant management* or *watchful waiting,* as if our therapeutic intervention is just being held temporarily at bay. Even in deciding to wait or do nothing, we imbue these periods with action. It is as if we are dynamically managing time and at the end of that time there may be more treatment for us to initiate.

We can confuse these interventions with hope, particularly at the end of life, and equate more treatment with more love. Any decision to hold or even withdraw treatment becomes near impossible, and not treating a patient the moral equivalent of giving up. Moreover, once treatments have started, there is an obligation to the interventions themselves. Having done so much already, doctors—and many patients and families—find it nearly impossible to let all their efforts simply drop.

In an attempt to display competency or undying love, we lose sight of the double-edged nature of our cutting-edge wizardry. We battle away until the last precious hours of life, believing that cure is the only goal. We inflict misguided treatments on not just others but also ourselves. During these final, tortured moments it is as if the promise of the nineteenth century has become the curse of the twenty-first.

You always know when there is a child undergoing surgery. Children easily become hypothermic after anesthesia has robbed them of their ability to shiver and surgeons have turned their insides out. The operating room, with its immaculately lined white tiles, spotless stainless steel surfaces, and sterile instruments, goes from feeling chilly, like a walk-in refrigerator, to oppressively hot, like an industrial steam room. Heating lamps that look like gawky french-fry warmers cluster around the operating table. Like observers anxiously peering into the field, the lamps insinuate their long metal necks and burning hot heads onto the napes and shoulders of the operating team.

Every time Max went to the operating room, the heat from those lamps got to me. While they blasted warmth down into Max's open belly, they also seemed to home in on the only exposed skin on my body, a small patch at the back of my neck. Initially, at the start of each of Max's operations, I welcomed this mechanical replacement for the sunshine I had not felt in days, working in basement operating rooms and insular intensive care units. By the end of each of Max's operations, however, as I whip-stitched the last blue nylon sutures through his ragged and raw skin edge, the heat from those insistent mechanical beings became a relentless reminder of the time spent working on this child.

Max was just a few months old when I first met him but already the tiny embodiment of a biological Keystone Kop. In utero, he had developed a gaping defect of his abdominal wall called gastroschisis, and the unprotected loops of his intestines slithered by one another in the open bath of his teenage mother's womb. While he was still in the middle of his third trimester of life, Max's intestines twisted around themselves, cutting off their own blood supply and becoming a gangrenous, necrotic mass of guts. The obstetricians delivered Max emergently via cesarean section, and the pediatric surgeons, waiting in another room with scalpels in hand, immediately removed the dead remnants of nearly his entire bowel.

When Max was four months old, his sixteen-year-old

mother, overwhelmed by her son's increasingly complicated care, relinquished custody of her baby. By the age of
eight months, Max had in quick succession experienced
every possible complication of total parenteral nutrition,
or TPN, the intravenous feeding he required to grow and
survive. Finally, Max's liver failed, the worst possible
complication from TPN. His liver stopped manufacturing
clotting factors, so the doctors' and nurses' needle pokes
bled without end. His warm brown complexion turned yellow, and he stopped kicking and smiling, lethargic from
the buildup of toxic by-products left unmetabolized by his
ailing liver. When he began to vomit blood regularly, small
bags of platelets, the cells that help clot, festooned his
crib-side like clusters of creamy-colored balloons.

At ten months Max received a liver and small bowel
transplant. The transplanted organs worked initially; he
stopped bleeding, squirmed in his bed, and even began to
grab at the objects around him. With a small feeding tube
inserted directly into his gut, Max digested for the first
time in his life tablespoons of food, albeit only a chalky
liquid supplement.

Within two months, however, Max again took up resi-
dence in the pediatric intensive care unit, wavering
between life-threatening infections and acute organ rejection. Achieving the right balance of immunosuppression
so he could keep the transplanted organs and yet maintain
sufficient immunity to fight off infection had become an
impossible task.

I was in my fellowship at the time of Max's transplant,
and Eric, an attending surgeon, was one of Max's primary
caretakers. A few years older than I, Eric led the surgical
team's management of Max's case. With a square jaw and
dark looks not unlike Dick Tracy's, Eric was a talented
young surgeon who had successfully transplanted other

young children. As Max became sicker, Eric would spend more hours with his tiny patient, bringing Max's records to his office to read whenever he couldn't be with Max. I found him by Max's bedside at 3:00 in the morning and then at 7:00 the next night, his hair, clothes, and personal aura in a state that reflected obliviousness to his own care. Just by being with Max so much, Eric knew every particularity of that baby, all his idiosyncratic reactions; he could recite every significant lab result of Max's entire life. Eric once said to me, "Max seems to be left-handed. Did you notice how he tends to flail with that arm?" I had not, and Eric reacted with surprise to my ignorance. "That's why the nurses keep his breathing tube turned toward the right," he went on, emphasizing, at least in my mind, that all those who really cared for Max knew about this left-handed business.

At first I found Eric's dedication inspiring, almost thrilling in a martyred-saint kind of way. And Max seemed to call out to any of us who hoped to be divinely touched. Before he had received the transplant, I had often absent-mindedly played with him to prevent myself from falling asleep during discussions on rounds. In an almost conspiratorial way, Max smiled at me, even giggled, as if he understood that playing with him was infinitely more interesting than arguing over doses of medication with other doctors. Spurred on by Max's cause, I found myself racing to uncover test results before Eric, as if my quicker response would translate into an equal or greater enthusiasm for Max's plight. I nagged the radiology technicians to give me Max's X-rays hot off the presses and then would smugly run with the still-warm films in my hands to the radiologists for a preliminary reading. I was determined to know the results first and thus come to Max's aid. I set the alarms on my beeper and asked the operators to page me at odd hours to remind me to check on Max. I wanted to see him in the middle of the night and on mornings long before the crack of dawn, before any member of the regular medical or surgical team, particularly Eric, arrived.

Every morning, as part of my maniacal routine, I examined Max in excruciating detail from head to toe. Coordinating my exam with the nurses' 6:00 a.m. dressing change, I pulled away every covering, gauze, tie, and wrap from Max's bloated torso. The bottommost layers were often heavy with the pink wetness that had seeped out from Max's belly since the last change four hours earlier. Gingerly removing that last layer, I could see our surgical work. Because Max had never developed an abdominal wall, we had sutured a thick piece of sterile white plastic to his sides to keep the new transplanted guts covered. When Max coughed, the plastic would bulge forward. With each strain the blue sutures holding the plastic to his flesh would pull through, adding a bloody pink color to the clear fluid that already oozed between the cracks.

As the weeks passed, despite my enthusiastic attentions, Max became sicker. Because his body kept trying to reject his transplanted organs, we gave Max high doses of steroids, and he quickly developed the characteristic ballooned-out cheeks of moon facies. His tiny body became engorged with fluid from repeated infections, and his big, shiny black eyes turned into a pair of hyphens on the rolling swells of his body. Sprawled out on the adult hospital bed necessary to accommodate all his medical machinery, Max had acquired enough equipment to require his own personal team for transport. He constantly needed a ventilator more than five times his size connected to a breathing tube whose diameter was not much bigger than a pencil. The tubing for his bladder was hardly fatter than a telephone wire, and it snaked from his bladder, out his urethra, and through the bloated head of his miniature penis, carrying droplets of urine to a bag that hung at the side of his bed.

Over the course of his ICU stay, Max's once buttery skin slowly became the ridiculously inadequate biological grounding for monitors and catheters. Several wires connected Max to a cardiac monitor; they were secured on his body with small circular adhesives that were covered with animal cartoons, as if such decoration would make all that wiring less frightening. Because there was not enough space on his person to hold everything, the nurses took to using the bed around him to clip wires and anchor dressings. They hung the mechanized pumps attached to his catheters on tall poles with wheels. Bigger, healthier kids in the hospital used these kinds of poles as modified skateboards, standing on top of the wheeled bases and pushing themselves down the length of the ward. For Max, however, the poles only served as another place to hang a piece of equipment, and they stood like skeletal beasts of burden crowded around the head of his bed.

Through all of Max's crises, Eric never let up. With every temperature spike came an acceleration in fervor from Eric. Even when he pulled himself away for a vacation, Eric called me almost relentlessly about Max, and the tone in his voice seemed to reproach the rest of us for not keeping up with Max as he would have. Eventually, not a single one of us dared write an order in Max's chart without first calling Eric, for fear that he might rail against us on rounds or begin a frantic series of pages on our beepers. A phone call would follow, as well as that inevitable question from the other end of the line: "What *were* you guys thinking?"

Despite Eric's most heroic efforts, Max was going to

die soon if we could not find the source of his ongoing infections. None of the X-rays showed anything suspicious in his belly, and with Max so sick already, an unnecessary trip to the OR and any accidental intraoperative mishap could send him over the edge. However, Eric finally decided to take Max to the operating room, fearful that the fevers were coming from a hidden pocket of infection around his transplanted intestines. "We've got to take him back to the OR," he said to us one afternoon on rounds. Eric looked at us, then asked rhetorically, "I mean, is there any other option?" We all understood what Eric was really asking. Were we doing enough? Was it *our* fault?

That trip to the OR would be the first of almost a dozen, and every return became a miserable mission. Under those searing heat lamps, we snipped the sutures that held the plastic patch in place and looked back into that small cavity filled with congealed organs. We picked away at the blocklike mass, edgy with a hyper-awareness of our Hippocratic pledge to do no harm. We were terrified of inadvertently cutting a hole in his transplanted intestine and creating another source of infection, yet we were afraid that if we did not search thoroughly enough, we might miss a hidden pocket of contamination. Then, finding nothing and too scared to cause any more damage, we put a new piece of plastic back over Max's belly. The suture we used handled like fine nylon fishing line, and we whipstitched the plastic to the edge of Max's abdominal wall. But after a half dozen operations, the edges of Max's belly became gangrenous and began to slough. It became harder and harder to find a square millimeter of untouched flesh where we could place a new stitch.

A little over a month later, Max died of a fungal infection that had managed to seep into his blood and into almost every organ system, including his brain. Later that day, when I was in the operating room for another case, I mentioned Max's death to the head operating room nurse. Jamie was a pragmatic woman, a brilliant nurse who possessed more insight into our patients and hospital politics than most of the physicians. She looked at me flatly when I told her the news, pausing for a moment and then returning to her work.

"Maybe it was a good thing, huh?" she said as she switched the suction tubing from one canister to another. She walked out of the room, and I could hear her asking aloud, "I mean, how much can you do to a person?"

For months after Max's death, I wondered about our collective role in his demise. I knew that Eric was a good doctor who cared immensely, heroically even, for Max. Eric had done everything for him and had even beat me in the race to be Max's most enthusiastic medical proponent. However, I could not shake the memories of that little baby's last month—his open abdomen, his raw and overworked skin, and the ever-present instruments of my profession.

In his helpless and voiceless state, Max was like an electron microscope that took our nearly invisible tangle of submerged responses and magnified them to the point where they took on lives of their own. We wanted to do everything for this child, and the pediatricians and we surgeons decided to use all the extremes of technology—a cluster transplant of liver and small bowel and the finest critical care available in the world—to do so. Even when we felt ambivalent about the extent of our efforts, we were unable to turn back or discuss and resolve these difficult feelings and differences among ourselves. Maybe we were doing too much to Max, but we had become bound to our technology. Pediatric-sized donor organs are rare, so the cost of losing Max would be not just his life but theoretically three lives in all: Max, the young donor, and another child on the transplant list who died waiting after Max had received the organs instead.

The pediatricians called up every medical treatment for Max, and my surgical colleagues and I soothed our own grief and helplessness with every trip to the operating room. We were trapped in a trajectory of our own making, and despite inklings of self-doubt, we continued to ascend along the interventional spectrum until we had made mincemeat out of the object of our care.

Doctors are not the only ones who find themselves in this kind of quandary. Patients and their families are equally susceptible to the intoxicating power of treatment. Patients now sometimes subject themselves to therapy in the belief that any kind of treatment may mean potential cure and is better than none. There is no more poignant and courageous example than patients who have enrolled in Phase I cancer trials. Phase I studies are the earliest trials and set out to examine an unproven treatment's maximum-tolerated dose and potential toxicity; Phase II and III studies determine whether that treatment will eventually yield results. Cancer patients enrolled in Phase I trials generally have later-stage tumors and only a few months' life expectancy; and while these trials are vitally important to the development of new therapies, less than 6 percent of patients enrolled will actually experience any kind of response to the treatment. Nonetheless, in two recent studies, the vast majority of Phase I candidates believed that they would benefit from such therapy. In one study patients believed they would live for two years or more with the experimental treatment. While this misunderstanding also reflects poor communication between the

Phase I investigators and patients, it reveals the inherent patient optimism regarding treatment and outcome. Simply put: if doing a little is good, then doing more must be better.

In this context, dying becomes a personal failure and withdrawing treatment the declaration of defeat. And pulling back therapy is even more difficult when there are unresolved personal issues for the physician or between the patient and family members. At the end of life the desire among patients and those around them to resolve past issues and to make things right is particularly strong, and there is no more apt stage upon which to play out these emotions than that of disease and treatment. Pushing for greater intervention is the seemingly natural extension of these feelings, and treatment becomes a metaphor not only for love but also for hope.

Nevertheless, even the most aggressive among us have an uneasy relationship with hope-driven treatment. Many doctors witness firsthand the painful, bungled results of a colleague's or their own technology-happy treatment decisions and see themselves as failing patients by overtreating. When asked what they would request for themselves if diagnosed with a terminal illness, the overwhelming majority of doctors choose to limit or withdraw life-sustaining therapy. These physicians are likely to support those patients who ask to withdraw care, but may feel obligated to continue treatment in others, for fear of legal repercussions.

These paradoxical impulses—to advocate treatment and to fear treatment outcomes—result in a difficult ethical angst. In a recent study, a third of the fully trained attending physicians and almost three quarters of the residents felt they had acted against their conscience in providing care to the terminally ill. More than half offered their patients mechanical ventilation, CPR, dialysis, artificial nutrition, and hydration, even as they believed those treatments to be "overly burdensome."

So how does one resolve these tangled webs? How do we, as physicians, families, and patients, know when to stop treating and begin palliating?

When I have asked that question of patients and my own family, their answer seems straightforward enough: stop treating when there is no more hope. From this point of view, the real issue then is not the decision but the explicit permission from the patient to stop treatment at the appropriate time.

That consent has been legally available in all fifty states since 1992 in the form of advance directives. However, only roughly a fifth of all Americans have prepared an advance directive, and there are wide discrepancies between different ethnic groups in the United States. White Americans, for example, are more likely than African Americans to draw up such legal documents.

And contrary to popular belief, advance directives do not ensure better end-of-life care: there are few differences between patients in terms of medical treatment and symptoms such as pain, agitation, and shortness of breath. I have seen patients and families come to the hospital with detailed advance directives in hand, but when faced with the reality of withholding treatment, they agonize. The same considerations made when drawing up these directives—most notably the prevention of suffering—come into play. Now, however, there is also the grief-ridden anticipation of loss and the nagging worry that death might be anticipated too quickly. Choices that seemed so clear-cut in a lawyer's office suddenly become morally and emotionally complicated, and decisions to withhold treatment are stalled by the hope that there might still be some time left. More than once, family members have told me that they do not want to be the one responsible for "pulling the plug." While directives do provide a framework for physicians and caregivers to follow, even the most detailed plans do not always fully prepare patients and families for the complex realities of dying.

There can also be significant differences between what patients and their loved ones or primary caregivers perceive as acceptable. With or without directives, families grapple with emotional issues and different notions of what constitutes a meaningful life. In one study, 46 percent of patient-caregiver pairs disagreed about the use of cardiopulmonary resuscitation, and 50 percent of them disagreed about the use of a respirator.

Physicians, too, may be poor judges of a patient's desires at the end of life. For example, physicians have widely varying interpretations of the DNR, or Do Not Resuscitate, order. Although the order specifies only that no resuscitative efforts be administered should the patient's heart stop, doctors and nurses may interpret DNR as a global shift of direction, easing up on *all* treatments, regardless. During my training, the news that a patient had "changed status" often came as a relief to residents; there was a sense that we suddenly had one fewer patient to care for.

Ultimately, the difficulty with "letting go" may have little to do with our inner struggles but may instead be wrapped around the ill-defined nature of dying. We have no reliable way of ascertaining when someone will die. Even with the best medical predictors—physician assessments and statistics—there is often a huge gap between perceived dying and the actual imminence of death. The accumulated scientific knowledge from Luke Fildes's lifetime onward has decelerated death's essential tempo, so that we have become less certain of when that final hurdle will be in front of us. Diseases that were once definitive precursors to death are now temporary inconveniences or even relatively minor annoyances. What finally then undermines the seemingly clear line of reasoning—stop treating when there is no more hope—is that death is no longer the self-contained time point we imagine it to be. It is a process.

And among our misperceptions of dying, it is this belief—that *death* is a certain, discrete event completely distinguishable from *life*—that cripples us most when we are deciding about end-of-life care. Doctors Joanne Lynn and Joan Harrold, in their book *Handbook for Mortals*, write:

> Perhaps the classification as "dying" is really more like height than it is like gender. Some people are clearly "tall" or "short," but many are "in between." Likewise, some people are clearly "dying" or "fully healthy," but many are "in between." In fact, most of us will die without having a period when we could readily be recognized as "dying" or "terminally ill." The new reality is that most of us will die from complications of a serious chronic illness that we will "live with" for years. There will only occasionally be a transition from that "living with" to a time of "dying from."

Perhaps all those scientific advancements have given us more than the panoply of treatments and longer life expectancies; they have created an impetus to reappraise how we live. By accepting the reality of dying rather than the misconception, we paradoxically give ourselves the luxury of time. The process of dying can be cast as full of potential rather than as devoid of any final opportunities. There is a chance for real interpersonal reconciliation and emotional expression rather than the hasty symbolic gesture of aggressive treatment.

It is this opportunity, then, and not necessarily the hope of cure, that is the final gift of the medical revolution of the last century.

The last time I saw Sam alert was about three weeks before he died from metastatic liver cancer. He had sent a donation in my honor for cancer research, and I went to visit him at his home a couple of days after receiving the gift. He was working with his physical therapist and was splayed out on a table as she led him through different exercises. Sam greeted me as he always did, with a slight nod of his head.

"How are you?" I asked him, holding his hand for a moment. He was dressed completely in white, from the tip of his padded athletic socks to the neckline of his loose mandarin shirt.

Sam rolled his eyes. "Pretty well, considering," he said. He swung his legs over to the side of the table and sat up. He lowered his voice to just above a whisper and leaned over to me. "I'm not going to last very long, am I? This tumor in my brain is just going to grow, isn't it?"

I nodded. Sam and Joanne had decided to stop all therapy, and we had talked about his prognosis at least twice before over the phone.

Sam released my hand and slid off the table so that he was standing next to me. He looked at me over his round spectacles.

"So you got it?" he asked. It took me a minute to realize that he was referring to his check.

"Yes," I replied. I had just finished my thank-you note earlier that morning. I was hoping that it would get to Sam before his tumor did. "Thank you. It was so generous."

Sam patted my hand and whispered, "Thank *you*." He padded away in his athletic socks and white outfit. "I'm going to go rest for a bit now," he said, his voice trailing off.

Sam remained alert for another week, and he and Joanne spent every minute together. They went to Nathan's, a sentimental favorite, for hot dogs and spent afternoons with friends and family. Sam also brought Joanne to the finest tuxedo store in Beverly Hills and proceeded to try on a dozen as his wife sat watching. "I have no idea why he did that," Joanne told me later. "It was just crazy. We had no functions to attend, and deep down I knew he would never wear it. But I kept quiet and went along and watched him try on every tuxedo and buy the most expensive one." Joanne sighed sadly. "It was as if he needed to reassure himself that he was alive. Maybe, just for a few moments, he wanted to believe that he was not going to die."

The last time I saw Sam, he was nearly comatose, breathing heavily and hardly able to speak. Christie, Sam's transplant case manager, and I had arranged hospice care, and the hospice nurse was at Sam's bedside when I arrived. Sam recognized my voice, held my hand, and thanked me once again for what I had done.

Sam died in his sleep at home with Joanne and his children by his side. A few days later there was a small private funeral followed by a large memorial service and reception in their home.

A week after the memorial service I went back to see Joanne. She looked better rested but no less sad. "I am trying to go through all of Sam's things," she said, walking me

through their closet and bedroom. She pointed to his side
of the closet. "My God, there is so much. He was such a
pack rat." She opened a box filled with watches. "Did you
know that Sam loved watches?" she asked me as she
picked up a couple and fingered over the rest in the collection. I looked at Joanne's forearm. A large oversized man's
watch dangled on her fine pale wrist. "I'm not sure what
I'm going to do with all of these watches," she said, looking down. "I mean, I can't wear all of them at once." She
opened the closet where the new tuxedo hung, still covered in the store's protective bag. "What am I going to do
with this now?" she asked me. "Do you think the store will
accept it as a return?"

As I prepared to leave, Joanne showed me a black-
and-white photo taken soon after their marriage. The photo
was stunning, like a *Life* magazine reprint. They are leaving a restaurant; Joanne is wearing a printed dress, the
wide skirt blooming out from her small waist, and Sam a
dark double-breasted suit. I caught my breath. There are
so many jasmine blossoms hanging from the awning that it
appears that someone has cast a net of white flowers
around the couple. And Sam and Joanne are smiling
broadly, walking forward and in step, hands locked
together.

Chapter 8 _____

SORRY TO INFORM YOU _____

I don't have a strong voice. It's one of those airy-sounding mid-rangers, the kind that gets crusty with the slightest overuse and that disappears the moment a cold virus materializes. When I speak to others, I am always trying to compensate for the lack of decibels, even if we are in the smallest of rooms. I sit directly in front of my audience and almost always begin by asking if they can hear me. I linger over consonants, pucker my lips around vowels, and then shift still closer.

There are certain conversations where, despite all these efforts, my voice fails me. I find myself gurgling over words and gulping for air through an ever-tightening throat. My voice comes out in breathy bursts, and I silently pray that my misery is not obvious.

Finally the words emerge, so softly that I see everyone leaning in as I speak. "I wonder," I hear myself saying to these people, "if you have thought of what you want at the end of life?"

I had my only lesson on talking with patients during my second year of medical school. Every Thursday, as part of an introductory skills course, a parade of specialists lectured to us on the patient exam. Although we were beginning to practice these skills on real patients once a week, we still spent six-hour days in the same lecture hall, taking notes on scores of disease and drug names, body parts, and biological pathways. We were starved for *real* doctor work, so the specialists who dropped their pearls of wisdom upon us were the enlightened, albeit eccentric, emissaries from the clinical world. A theatrical bearded cardiologist rolled his eyes and sprayed saliva onto the lecture hall microphone as he imitated the lub-dubs and whooshes of a heart; a pasty pulmonologist, his cheeks puffing out and turning blue, whistled and wheezed for us; and a dermatologist, whose own epidermis appeared very much stretched over her long frame, introduced a new language with words that rolled off our tongues: "erythematous," "macular," "papules."

One of the last lectures that first semester was "The Patient Interview." Compared to ones divulging the secret signs and language of illness, this topic struck me as nearly superfluous. Conversing with patients seemed like an obviously natural skill, one that hardly required an hour's instruction. Nevertheless, with final exams coming up, I was happy to have fluff, not more facts, fill an hour of the day.

The lecturer was an oncologist in the medical center, known for her compassionate work with the terminally ill. She was tiny, barely five feet, with sparkling eyes and a mouth filled with brilliant straight white teeth. Her brown hair was unusually short, cropped so that there were only a few wisps around her ears and neck. One of my classmates leaned over to me just as her lecture was about to begin. "She has breast cancer, you know." I looked up. The lecturer seemed as healthy as any of us, and with her smile and petite height, she looked a good deal younger than any of the previous lecturers. "Chemo," the classmate whispered to me again, and I suddenly understood the sparseness of her hair.

The lecturer turned down the room lights. "I want to start with a movie." Her voice was clear and surprisingly strong. "You'll see two different examples of the patient interview," she continued. "I know these are kind of corny, but I think you will get the point."

The first half of the movie featured a balding male doctor. He sat stiffly in his chair and asked such abrupt questions of his patient that my classmates and I could hardly stifle our laughs. The second half of the movie showed a more relaxed and handsome doctor who smiled and stopped writing to look at the patient whenever he asked a question.

When the short movie ended, the lecturer turned the hall lights back on. "Can you tell me which doctor has the better interview technique?" she asked. We laughed, and the lecturer flashed her sparkling smile. "Note that the second doctor asked open-ended questions," she said. "It's really important to allow your patients to speak and be listened to." She walked to the blackboard and asked us to name important interview techniques. She wrote a few of our answers:

1. Ask open-ended questions.
2. Listen.
3. Look at your patient.

Then she added a few of her own:

4. Don't talk at your patient.
5. Ask them why they came in to see you.
6. Figure out how they perceive their medical
   problems.

As she wrote on the blackboard, I looked around the lecture hall. Everyone, despite the occasional laughter, looked bored, and one student in the last row had fallen asleep. His head was cocked back; his mouth hung open.

The lecturer put her chalk down. "What's the take-home lesson, then, folks?" she asked. She walked to the edge of the stage, where the overhead lights shone brightest. Leaning forward, she looked as if she were about to fall into the audience. The lights reflected off her hair, and the gray strands were suddenly visible. "If you remember anything from today, I want you to remember this." Her smile disappeared, and her dark eyes looked as if they had suddenly pooled with water.

"You'll be a better doctor," she said, "if you can stand in your patients' shoes."

The entire class fell silent. But it was *not* because this woman, who was both doctor and patient, had moved us; it was because we believed that her statement went without saying. Most of us viewed ourselves as different from the old guard, *her* generation of physicians, those wise but hopelessly odd fuddy-duddies who made strange noises into the class microphone to imitate their organ of choice or who showed bloody clips from their latest operation or who droned on and on about the specific pathways of disease on which they had staked their clinical reputations.

I certainly believed my classmates and I were destined for something different. Sure, we had yet to learn practical skills in our training, but that did not affect our confidence in the future. Unlike those before us, we had been raised to question the old patriarchal doctorly ways: what would set *us* apart would be our willingness to listen to patients. Already during our weekly interviews with practice patients, we were able to write novellas recounting every detail of the patients' lives, including facts they had never even shared with their regular physicians. And somehow, naïvely enough, we believed that our teachers had never been able to do the same.

After that lecture was over, none of us ever talked about "The Patient Interview" again. Some of us saw the lecturer working in the hospital and remembered the movie. Others passed by her and wondered about her cancer. I went for a dozen years, through internship, residency, and two fellowships, before I thought of her again.

And when she popped back into my mind, she was back on that stage. Despite my early hubris, conversing with patients was not a skill that would appear effortlessly. Unlike auscultating lungs or a heart or describing a skin rash, all of which eventually became second nature, learning to converse with patients was not a skill that came with practice. It became, in fact, more difficult and elusive with time. And it was only at the very end of my training, during moments I found nearly unbearable, that I finally remembered that lecturer and her advice: to be a good doctor, I had to stand in my patients' shoes.

. . .

My younger sister, Lena, works at a busy academic medical center. A fully trained attending in internal medicine, she is a hospitalist, a physician whose clinical practice consists of overseeing and directing the course of care of hospital inpatients. Lena recently asked a medical specialist at her hospital to see a patient. There are unspoken rules of etiquette among physicians; we try to remain polite and collegial to one another, particularly during consultations such as these, when your practice as a specialist is as dependent on how you treat the referring doctor as on how you care for the patient.

Lena called the specialist and briefly described her patient's problem. Expecting the usual—"Thanks for this interesting consultation! I'll see the patient as soon as I can!"—she was taken aback by the doctor's response. The specialist berated my sister, dressing her down as if she were a medical student or intern. When Lena began to reproach the consultant for lack of professionalism, the woman backed off, saying, "Listen, I am not having a good day. I am stuck in clinic still, and I have a lot of bad news to tell some patients, so I am stressed out and probably won't go to see your patient."

I have to give that specialist some credit. She was, unlike some of us, extraordinarily self-aware. Short on time and behind on work, she was having a terrible day. And it was only made worse by the prospect of difficult patient discussions: she, with bad news in hand, was going to be responsible for the abrupt disintegration of another person's life. Even writing about the situation now, I cannot help but feel sorry for her.

Almost every doctor has been there, and it's a horrible place to be. The common thread running through our professional world is disease, and many of our conversations inevitably converge on "bad news." They may begin with an initial diagnosis, but those diseases can become cata-strophic or just sputter along in a continuous decline until death. We doctors must be there every step of the way. Bad news thus occurs not just once but over and over again.

As a resident watching my attending surgeons deliver bad news, I believed that practice would make perfect. Eventually, over time, I would know how to word terrible news in sympathetic ways, be gentle in my delivery, and finish off with an appropriately uplifting note. But these conversations never got easy—not for me, nor for almost anyone else. Medical oncologists, for example, work with cancer patients, a fair percentage of whom do not get definitively cured. One would assume, then, that oncolo-gists get pretty good at talking with patients about difficult topics. A recent study, however, revealed that more than a quarter of oncologists failed to tell their patients that they had incurable cancer.

Like the miserable specialist who spoke rudely to my sister, many physicians are also probably keenly aware of their failure in this regard. In another study, again of oncologists, almost half of the doctors rated themselves as only "poor" to "fair" when it came to breaking bad news to their patients. To compensate for this failure, doctors may deny the reality of their patients' condition and push for more therapy right up to and through the most terminal stages of a disease.

Several factors compound this difficult situation. The health care system has become highly specialized; conse-quently, a single patient can have multiple subspecialty physicians. With half a dozen doctors responsible for as many body parts, it is impossible for a patient and the physicians to know which doctor is responsible for initiat-ing the more global discussions about prognosis and death. In the case of my college roommate's father, it was not the oncologist or the primary care doctor who spoke to him that one time about dying; it was a consulting specialist in pulmonary medicine. With individual responsibilities so ill-defined, physicians can—almost without realizing it—completely bypass these difficult conversations.

Up until more recently, there were few internal systems of accountability for situations like these. Since most physicians were wary of the dying to begin with, there was little to counter the inclination to evade these topics. However, as more professional organizations and state licensing boards incorporate end-of-life care into their requirements, and as medical educators push to broaden the scope of conferences such as M and M, this situation may change. Initiating these difficult conversations will no longer be dependent on a clinician's personal sense of responsibility but will become part of a well-defined and well-promulgated professional code of conduct.

Another complicating factor is the enormous variation in patient responses to bad news. Some patients want to hear the information with cool scientific objectivity; others prefer gentle counseling and a human touch. Some patients associate these topics with cultural stigmas; and others, in an attempt to appear dignified, conceal feelings and fears even as they are becoming increasingly impaired. I have had to discuss bad news in rooms bursting with weeping, grieving family members and in rooms so silent that I could hear the tape recorder roll as I answered questions about the current data on disease outcomes.

One year out from my internship, I told a family that their sixteen-year-old son, who had become intoxicated and fallen into a pool during a party, might be brain-dead. In that small family conference room in the middle of the night, the mother heard only the term "brain-dead." A week later, when her son recovered partially—his cognitive functions still severely compromised but working enough so that he no longer required a ventilator—she trailed me every time she saw me in the halls, yelling that I was the "fraud doctor" who had declared her son brain-dead. In retrospect, the fault was mine, for I failed to gauge my audience and to understand that this mother would shut down after hearing "brain-dead." Any discussion about nuances of recovery would, along with this mother's sense of hope, disappear. Her son never did leave the hospital; he died three weeks later after a cardiac arrest.

For doctors, responding appropriately to any given patient is at best extraordinarily challenging and at worst extremely time-consuming. And time in the hospital is *the* most precious of commodities. As an intern and resident, I worked fourteen-hour days and was awake through every other or every third night. I had no time to stand in someone else's shoes; I could barely remember what *my* shoes looked like.

I left my home at 5:00 a.m. to prepare for work rounds at 6:00 a.m. and then worked on patient tasks— scheduling the tests, gathering the results, writing the orders, contacting the consultants, cleaning the wounds, changing the dressings, visiting the consultations, seeing the patients in clinic, doing the bedside procedures, discussing patient care plans with the attending surgeons— until I would have temporary respite in the form of operating on a patient. When that operation was over, I scrambled out to catch up on lost time, picking up pieces as I had left them or, as was more often the case, running to put out the clinical fires that had ignited in my hours away.

The patients on my surgical service, twenty to thirty as a resident and up to seventy as a fellow, were rarely stable; surgery as a specialty is acute care at its most urgent. And with the constant stream of clinical and operative demands and the never-ending supply of new patients from the emergency room and other wards of the hospital, I learned that exhaustion leaves its own olfactory imprint. The white coats of residents who had been up through the night had an acrid, stale odor—the smell of dirtied polyester, sweat-stained cotton, and human flesh trapped too long away from sunlight and normal circadian rhythms. I could recognize my exhausted colleagues with my eyes closed.

I believed that all these work hours would turn me into a well-trained surgeon, but in the heat of the everyday moment that lofty goal rarely entered my thoughts. Instead, it was anxiety that pervaded my days. My unquestioning acceptance of the training and the work hours was driven by a single fear: that I might otherwise make *the* mistake that could *kill* someone. The thought shadowed me constantly, and like some indestructible umbilical cord, it tethered my mind to the hospital. It drove me to wake up on nights away from the hospital and to sift through my papers to see if I had done everything correctly. It made me call the hospital during my days off to check up on things.

And it changed the way I talked to patients.

Whenever I was trapped in some patient's room, I could feel the next clinical task pushing at me. I wanted to keep moving; only when standing could I feel the burden of the day's scut list in my white coat pockets. Halfway through a sentence, I would begin to edge toward the patient's door, impelled to start moving again lest I become permanently anchored to the room. Instead of getting better at talking to patients, I became expert at cutting conversations short.

And a few months into my internship, I glommed on to one of the oldest tricks of the resident trade, a maneuver that would, when all else failed, trim my load of responsibilities. I learned how to "turf," to send difficult, time-consuming problems to someone else. Patients with chronic problems could go to the internists; those with a few lingering medical issues could go to rehabilitation. I would not have to face my medical failures—patients who were still unable to go home because of their disease or, worse yet, who suffered from some debilitating complication of surgery. Granted, many of these transfers were medically appropriate, but to me they felt like welcome releases of responsibility.

In the case of patients who had no apparent medical reason to leave me, such as those who needed to be told bad news, I found an even more creative way of turfing. I evaded the issue altogether, convincing myself that some other, more experienced member of the team would eventually pick up on the responsibility. I knew that someone had to tell these patients about the terrible diagnosis or disheartening prognosis—that was what I would have wanted if our roles were reversed—but I knew that if I held off long enough, someone else probably would.

Turfing seemed the ideal remedy. It was ingenious and completely subconscious. I did not have to lie, and I did not have to divulge the truth. I did not have to see the smiles drop nor be the one to put the pin to my patients' enormous bubble of hope. In one circuitous loop of thought, I could eliminate the problem from my own vista.

But the fact that I could not muster the strength to tell the truth to these patients sickened me. I continued to care for them—cheery greetings every morning and upbeat plans for the day's scheduled studies—yet as I walked away, I always felt that same twisting of my gut, as if something I had swallowed had long gone bad.

By the time I entered the last year of my transplant fellowship, turfing had become a part of my doctoring repertoire. As far as any patient conversation was concerned, I had convinced myself that I was still providing the most competent of care but just letting someone else deliver part of it. I was, after all, just the surgeon and not—or so I thought—someone who needed to linger in the shoes of the dying.

Lou was the kind of nurse who should have been the doctor. Five feet and a little more if you included the thick wooden clogs she always wore, Lou had exuberant, dark curly hair, darting brown eyes made even rounder by her circular wire glasses, and neat but luxuriant eyebrows. As one of the nurse coordinators for the liver transplant team, she attended morning and afternoon work rounds, monitoring each of the inpatients and coordinating their eventual discharges.

Lou took some getting used to. She could be blunt and nearly relentless in her persistence; but what was most disarming—particularly to the surgical trainees—was her sharp intelligence, which she carried like a beautiful jewel that dazzled and blinded and held you utterly in awe. I used to think of her as a kind of quality-control bulldog. We had a gargantuan service of almost seventy patients, and part of the art of running that service was rounding on every patient in two and a half hours or less. The small group of residents and nurses led by the fellow would fly through the wards pushing a rack filled with charts and reports, their breezy course interrupted by perfunctory one-minute visits with the patients.

What Lou did so artfully on those lightning rounds

was patient advocacy in its most in-your-face form. Whenever her inner radar sounded after a less-than-satisfactory discussion about a patient, Lou would plant herself in front of the offending nurse or doctor and bring those quickly moving eyes to rest on her opponent. Her usual comments—"How come you are doing that?" or "What do you think about that lab abnormality, *Doctor*?"—seemed simple but were laden with meaning and implication. By the time the doctor or nurse realized something had been overlooked, Lou had all but backed her victim into the wall. It was very effective, and for those who witnessed Lou in action, it could even be fairly entertaining.

I was slightly surprised, then, when one day Lou pulled me aside after morning work rounds. We had worked together for almost two years, and under Lou's and the other nurses' guidance, I had learned to sharpen my own clinical skills under the time constraints of the service. Lou rarely questioned me anymore.

"Pauline, I want to talk to you about a patient," she said. Lou did her plant maneuver in front of me and looked directly into my eyes. I could see the reflection of the hall's fluorescent lights against her glasses. Old self-protective instincts began to rise immediately in my chest as I started to run through all the recent clinical issues. Was there some decision I had made that might have been a little less than solid?

"Do you remember Bobby?" she asked.

Of course I remembered Bobby. I had met Bobby a year and a half earlier, during my fellowship, when he came to our clinic with a large bile duct cancer in his liver. The cancer, a cholangiocarcinoma, had developed as a complication of a chronic inflammatory condition in his colon, ulcerative colitis, that he had had since he was fifteen. Lou had known Bobby for years from her previous work with the doctors who took care of his colon disease. A year earlier, after I had met Bobby for the first time in our surgical clinic, Lou specifically paged me to talk about her former patient. "Bobby is really a special person," she said. "Please take good care of him."

Bobby was thirty years old at the time and had spent his entire adult life enduring the peripatetic course of his disease. During a colitis exacerbation he would suffer from frequent, painful abdominal cramping and unremitting voluminous diarrhea. Inevitably, because of the severity of both, Bobby would have to interrupt school, or later, his work, and check in to the hospital for intravenous nutrition to renew his strength and for huge doses of intravenous steroids to quell the inflammation. Despite his malnourished state, Bobby's weight and face would balloon up from the steroids, and he often left the hospital looking, he liked to say, "like a big ol' chipmunk."

When I walked into the exam room to meet him for the first time, I expected a long and possibly painful encounter with an anxious young patient and his family. A week earlier I had met a nineteen-year-old boy who also had ulcerative colitis and developed the same cancer, and the softly spoken, angst-ridden pleas of his mother were still alive in my mind.

Bobby was seated on the examining table in the center of the small room. The venetian blinds in the exam room were partially opened, angled so that the bright afternoon sun of Los Angeles hit the white linoleum floor and then radiated upward around Bobby in a halolike glow. He appeared youthful, with smooth skin and a hearty round face. His mother and his fiancée, Chris, sat beside him, and because the sun was shining against their backs and into my face, their expressions appeared hazy, almost softened, the natural angles of their features totally obscured to my line of sight.

I steadied myself in front of this vision and began to

ask Bobby about his life and the crippling symptomatic episodes. He was an accountant, having graduated from high school and then college with honors. He was devoted to his church and had met Chris through the choir. They had just finished a choir tour together and were preparing for Chris's daughter's entry into a statewide youth talent pageant. Bobby pulled out photos of the young girl, showing them off to me as if we were old college buddies catching up on intervening years.

Bobby's tumor was large and located in the center of his liver; his operation turned out to be difficult. Even with my surgical mentor's prodigious surgical skills, we teetered dangerously between taking out too much liver or leaving cancer cells behind. Nonetheless, Bobby, with his characteristic understated grace, recovered from our high-tech marauding and, after a couple of postoperative visits to our clinic, was discharged from our care. He began seeing a medical oncologist for chemotherapy and continued to go to Lou's old work haunt, the inflammatory bowel disease clinic, for his ulcerative colitis.

About four months after Bobby's operation, Chris stopped by our clinic to show us her wedding ring while Bobby was seeing his medical oncologist. She told us that Bobby was tolerating everything. "He's cancer-free," she said in a whisper, as if saying it any louder might jinx the outcome. But a few months later Chris came by again to tell us that the oncologists were changing the chemotherapy. Though the tumor had returned, both she and Bobby were optimistic and believed he would be fine. After that visit I never saw Chris again.

Six months later Lou cornered me while I was making rounds. Bobby was back in the hospital, admitted to the medical service with complications from end-stage cancer. His cholangiocarcinoma had not only returned but had also spread to his lungs. Lou asked me to go to the medical floors to speak to Bobby and his wife about palliative options.

I agreed but then never went. The medical doctors who had admitted Bobby would take care of it, I thought.

Two weeks passed. Lou pulled me aside again from rounds and told me that Bobby was now in the intensive care unit, hooked up to a ventilator and a dozen monitors. She urged me again to talk to Bobby's wife, but I found other work to do.

I remembered all of this when Lou brought up Bobby again that morning. I looked down at Lou and noticed that she was pulling back away from me. When she looked up at me again, I could see a moist film over her eyes. I saw a tear forming, the rounded drop rolling over her lower eyelid and trickling down her cheek.

"Bobby died, you know," Lou said. She bit her lip and flicked away the tear with a finger. Lou put her hand on my arm. "He was dying, Pauline. He had cancer everywhere, and they still poked him and prodded him and thumped on his chest when he coded. They did the full-court press." Lou's lips became thin. She put her index finger against my chest and rapped it with each word. "That is how Bobby died."

Lou never brought Bobby up again. She never asked me why I had not gone to see him before he died. I was grateful to her for that, but I could not help asking that question of myself. I went to look for his medical records to piece together those last days, but most of Bobby's chart was missing, tied up in the hospital paperwork bureaucracy because of his recent death. I scanned the hospital computer records for physician dictations, but found only an admission note that mentioned Bobby's metastatic cancer and a recent CAT scan. I walked into the medical intensive care unit where Bobby had died, but could find no one who had taken care of Bobby or who might have known him as more than "the kid who died of cancer in Bed 7." I walked over to see where Bobby had spent his last days, but found in Bed 7 an elderly woman whose body was failing from a lethal urinary tract infection.

In the end I could only turn to two images of Bobby. One was clear, as it was what I remembered so well: Bobby is sitting in my clinic exam room and I am basking in the unswerving faith of him and his relatives. The other was blurry, existing only in the darkness of my imagination: Bobby is lying unconscious, attached to and pinned down by the machinery of my profession.

For months, the disconnect between these two images prevented me from forgetting Bobby or from neatly filing him away in my "former patients" mental files. I kept wondering what would have happened if I had gone to see him. Maybe he would not have gone to the ICU. Maybe he would not have suffered in the end. Maybe he would have had the kind of death he deserved.

The old-time Taiwanese believed that certain souls haunt the world, searching for mollification for their untimely or dishonorable deaths. These *wan ong kuei*, "wronged spirits," are destined to wander among humans for eternity. Without any justification for his manner of death, Bobby became a *wan ong kuei* of my mind.

It was after Bobby died that I began choking on my words whenever I spoke to patients about dying.

In one of the professional journals I subscribe to, I recently came across yet another study that examined the effectiveness of workshops that train physicians how to engage in difficult conversations. I find these studies interesting, in part because I have often entertained the idea of submitting myself to such an experiment. Would my choking and gasping disappear if I learned these skills?

As in previous studies, these researchers found that the intense workshops could improve skills and that patients and physicians benefited from this training. What struck me most in reading through this study, however, was not the effectiveness of such courses but the sheer difficulty of getting doctors to participate. Out of the 214 physicians who were phoned, 3,706 who were invited by mail, and 2,741 who were contacted by an internal institutional letter of invitation, only 63 eventually completed the program. That's a recruitment rate of less than 1 percent; the researchers probably would have had just as much success if they had waited for participants to fall from the sky. And the greatest reason for refusal was not lack of interest but lack of time. In the grand schedule of things, improving difficult conversational skills was just not important enough. Or, as a doctor friend of mine put it, "Who has got the time?"

Time takes on exaggerated forms for physicians. There is, for example, the burden of the second. In certain instances, a patient's outcome—a baby in the birth canal whose umbilical cord has prolapsed, a man whose heart has stopped, a ventilator-dependent woman who has lost her tracheostomy—can take a devastating turn for the worse in a matter of a few seconds. Even in the least urgent of situations, the routine clinic visit, time gets no larger than the minute. Visits and all that they encompass— exam, treatment plan, and discussion—are scheduled in minutes: fifteen to twenty minutes for return visits, forty-five for new patients. In that context, five minutes devoted to talking about any topic is enormous.

Physicians have tried for years to find ways to respond to the pressures of time. Recently, they have focused on the worst time crunch in a physician's professional life: residency. Over the last five years, training programs, and most dramatically surgical ones, have enforced work-hour limitations in an effort to decrease sleep deprivation, improve quality of life, and, presumably, enhance patient care. While residents these days do spend less time in the hospital than those who trained even a decade ago, the change has had some unpredictable repercussions. The increased "free time" has left residents with less time to form bonds with their patients. The pressure now is to squeeze as much experience as possible into the time limitations, usually at the expense of patient relationships. The transient physician-patient relationships of residency have only become more fleeting. As one surgical resident said to me, "Definitely, as the hours get shorter, the premium on spending what time you do have in the OR gets higher, so patient time probably goes down."

This constant tension from the growing list of clinical tasks, the lack of time to perform them well, and the inability to have real conversations with patients leave physicians at all levels in a quandary. Renée Fox, a noted medical sociologist, has said, "Doctors' anguish seems to come from violating every day what they know they ought to be doing. The pain is from the degree to which they still espouse values but can't live up to them." A terrible sequence unfolds: the physician is constrained by time, chooses to winnow away less "urgent" responsibilities such as difficult patient conversations, feels increasingly worse for doing so, then ultimately burns out.

A group of researchers recently looked at burnout in more than 1,500 physicians in the United Kingdom from the start of medical school until ten years later. They discovered that certain personality traits were protective against professional burnout, while others were predictive of eventual disillusionment with work. Physicians who were more extroverted and open to new experiences tended to fare better and to complain of less stress than their counterparts. While these personality traits may be inborn, the researchers state, "just as genes are not destiny, so neither personality nor learning style is destiny." And just as many an introvert has trained to become a magnificent actor or public speaker, physicians can acquire the traits that avert burnout.

There is solace for my profession in those findings. But what is required is seeing ourselves and the work we do in an entirely different light.

It had been our private joke, a line that we repeated every time we saw each other in the halls and were reminded of how much we missed home. Frank, a strapping seventy-five-year-old Mediterranean Cary Grant, and I would intone the words together: "Mr. Martin lost a button in New Britain." With our strongest Connecticut Yankee accents and between the precipices formed by our gulped T's, Mr. Mar'in suddenly became inebriated, staggering about New Bri'ain, looking for that lost bu'on.

Frank had spent most of his life in a working-class burg in the northern part of Connecticut, just a few minutes from where I grew up. Soon after he retired as chief of police, his wife of forty years passed away, and Frank moved to the West Coast to be with his three grown children. But Frank, like me, remained nostalgic about his New England roots. Even during his first clinic visit, we could not help, much to the distress of the harried nurses and waiting patients, waxing lyrical about the gorgeous

New England autumns, tubing on the Farmington River, and the Shad Derby, my hometown's yearly celebration of fish come home.

Frank had a habit of treating others, including nurses, doctors, and patients, as if he were still the local police chief and the rest of us part of his protected constituency. He approached each person with a wide, toothy smile, his broad prominent cheekbones lending an aura of mischief and sex appeal. He extended his massive, well-padded hands and offered handshakes that left their imprint on your memory long after he had gone off to greet his next constituent. Even those who resisted these maneuvers inevitably became sucked into the vortex of Frank's charm once he began one of his yarns about past police escapades. Frank's persona delighted others and, I have often later thought, it gave him the strength to navigate his homesickness, his grief over losing his life partner, and the difficulties of his diagnosis.

Frank had a cholangiocarcinoma the size of a Ping-Pong ball. After hearing about chemotherapy and the response rate of 15 percent or less, Frank told his primary care physician that he was not interested. "I want to see a surgeon," he told his doctor. "I want to know if they can cut this thing out."

From a purely technical point of view, his tumor seemed entirely operable; we could remove it in a couple of hours. What concerned my surgical mentor and me, however, was that Frank had a fierce jaundice. The tumor was likely obstructing one of his bile ducts, and his jaundice was severe and long-standing enough to have crippled his liver. The first afternoon we met, Frank glowed like a yellow firefly. And, as I could tell from the small bloodstains under his fingernails, his biliary obstruction was making him itch miserably.

Our plan would be to ask the radiologists to insert a tube that would drain Frank's bile to the outside. The drainage would ameliorate his symptoms, but there was still a 30 percent chance that his liver would fail after an operation. His only option at that point would be transplantation.

"Would I get a transplant?" Frank asked me. He wore a white cotton sweater and, despite the jaundice, looked more like a movie star who had walked off the Los Angeles streets than a retired cop from Connecticut. He was smiling.

"No," I said. I looked down at the floor; I did not want to see his response to my answer. "You are a hair too old," I whispered.

"So I could die?" he asked.

I nodded.

Frank was silent for a moment. I heard him shifting in his chair and then felt his large hand on my shoulder. "Listen, Doctor," he said as I looked up, "I'm going to die from this thing. I know that. But I don't want chemo. I don't want to just sit around and wait to die." Frank's smile had disappeared, and his brown eyes had lost their glimmer. He looked at me. "I've thought about this, Doc. I've thought of nothing else since I heard about this tumor. I want the operation—whatever the risks—because I can't see there being any other way. I want to die giving it my best."

I began to list all the risks and benefits of operating. I wanted to make sure that Frank knew *all* the possible outcomes. He stood up, straining, it seemed, under the weight of my words. "I believe you, Doc. I really do, and I hear what you're telling me. There's a good chance I won't make it, but I *need* to do this." He paused and looked toward the window of the exam room.

"You'll be with me, right?" he asked.

Patients often asked me that question. Of course I would be with them; I was one of their surgeons. But I was also in training, and I *had* to be at the hospital all the time.

I nodded, and Frank smiled at my response. He straightened his shoulders and shook his head like a bull readying itself for the charge. "I'm ready, then," he said, taking my hand in that magnificent handshake of his. "As long as I have my Connecticut doctor, I am ready to take this operation on." He stepped out of the exam room, now grinning widely. "Let's get on with it!"

Frank's surgery did go well; we got the tumor out. And for the first couple of days after his operation, his recovery was uneventful. He got out of bed, sat up in a chair, and took a few steps around the room. But then, on his third postoperative day, his liver blood test results began to rise. They continued to worsen, as if the liver cells had become explosive biological dominoes falling down and fanning out in rapid succession. Within days Frank began to complain about trouble breathing, and his belly started to bloat with fluid.

I visited Frank twice a day. "Your liver took a bit of a hit, Frank," I said at each visit. "We need to try to nurse it back." I felt like the coach halfheartedly bolstering the spirits of a losing team. Frank's children, frequent visitors, even cheered every time they heard my words. Frank would only nod, and over time his response became groggier. His smile dulled, the corners of his lips sagged, and I would find him in his bed with eyes glazed over and mouth hanging slightly open.

I continued, however, to rally the team on.

Nine days after his operation, on one of his better

days, Frank motioned to me to sit next to him. I sat at the edge of his bed, and he put his hand in mine.

"You got it all out, didn't you?" he asked. His eyes were sharper than they had been but still looked slightly filmy.

I nodded. "The pathology report said that all the margins were clear of tumor."

"That's great," Frank replied slowly. He closed his eyes and then asked quietly, "Doc, how am I doing?" He squeezed my hand; those beautiful Cary Grant cheekbones jutted out sharply beneath his loose skin. I heard his daughter behind me, trying to muffle high, hiccoughed sobs; she sounded like an injured bird.

"Frank," I said. His opened his eyes, and his gaze slowly drifted over to me. I felt the familiar tightening around my throat. Thoughts rumbled around in my chest, like acidic, gaseous bubbles. I opened my mouth; the words popped out and hung in the air. "Your liver is struggling," I said.

Frank nodded. I had told him the obvious.

But Frank's liver was not struggling; it was failing. I knew that in the next few days he would likely fall into a coma and die. As I sat next to him, the inevitable repeatedly playing in my mind, I could not bring myself to describe that outcome. Instead, I wished to melt away and find myself back in that time before I had met Frank, when being homesick simply meant a place and a distant memory and not the shared joke and camaraderie with a patient whose death I felt all but responsible for. As I sat there, I wanted to forget my promise to stay with him, to erase my commitment to be his surgeon, and to take back the operation I had performed.

Instead, I said, "Well, let's just see how the numbers look tomorrow."

Frank looked at me. "I'm not going back to New Britain anytime soon, am I?"

"I don't think so, Frank," I said quietly. "I am so sorry."

Frank smiled, more radiantly than he had in days. "Doc, you did your best," he said slowly, "and I am grateful. Like I told you, if I'm going to go, this is the way I want it to happen." He took my hand and with a force that surprised me, pulled me close to his face. I could smell the spoiled sweetness of his breath. "Just keep me comfortable," he whispered. He squeezed my hand and as he let go, repeated the words once more. "Just keep me comfortable."

For the next week I forced myself to continue to visit Frank twice a day. I watched his consciousness slip away, his family members become more and more enveloped in their grief, and my voice dwindled in their presence to breathy whispers. When I was with Frank, I wanted nothing more than to leave; and when I was away from him, I thought of nothing but home. My mind wandered back to Connecticut, to his hometown, where I could smell the crisp scent of autumn, see the streets dappled with sunlight filtered through the colored leaves, and all but feel the welcoming backslaps of Frank's old colleagues celebrating his return. I would lose myself in these mental wanderings and then, when I pulled myself out, rush to return to Frank's room, to make sure he was comfortable, to make sure that he—far from home—was not alone.

Just over two weeks after his operation, Frank died. I went to his room minutes after he passed away; his three grown children and their spouses, all exhausted, surrounded his bed. "I need to pronounce his death," I said. They nodded, and I heard myself add, "May I have a few minutes alone with Frank?"

One by one, they embraced me as they left the room. When they closed the door, I half expected Frank's charisma to reignite, but the room remained dark and so silent that I could hear my own breathing. Frank's eyes were closed. His body, already pale, was perfectly still; his lips were slightly parted and pale blue; and his cheeks were sunken and unmoving, weighing down against those glorious arches of bone.

I knew the steps I had to perform—listen to the heart, listen to the lungs, pinch the flesh—but I could not bring myself to do it. Instead, I pulled up a chair and sat and waited, watching him, hoping he would open his eyes, flash that grin, and begin recounting Mr. Martin's misadventures with his buttons. I looked down at Frank's hands; they were now whitish, and his fingers were frozen in a gentle curl. I took his right hand and held it; it wasn't so cold yet. I wanted to feel his grasp and to hear him tell me again that this was how he had wanted it.

I fell back in my chair, wanting desperately for the tears to come forth to release the ache. But nothing came, nothing except for a faint rim of wetness around my eyes, easily dabbed dry with my fingers.

Six months later I received an envelope from Frank's daughter; she enclosed a letter, a photograph of Frank, and a small remembrance card from his memorial service in Connecticut. *I'm sorry that it's taken me so long to send this,* she wrote in her letter. *My father was so fond of you, and it was your spirit that gave him the strength to be himself in the worst of situations.*

The picture of Frank was from before I had met him, of a younger, more robust man with the same smile. On one side of the remembrance card was the date of Frank's service; on the other side, a poem he had chosen several years before. As I read through the poem, I heard Frank's voice grow stronger in my mind until, at the very end, each line lurched from the staccato of that familiar accent.

So if you need me, call and I will come.
Though you can't see or touch me, I'll be near.
And if you listen with your heart,
You'll hear my love around you soft and clear.
And then, when you must come this way alone,
I'll be waiting with a smile and say, "Welcome Home."

I put the card down and felt a sudden wave of relaxation across my arms, surging up to my throat. It felt as if the cartilaginous rings around my trachea loosened for a moment and great breaths of air could at last pass through. I opened my mouth, releasing the *wan ong kuei*, and in the quiet of my office, began to cry.

Chapter 9

THROUGH THE LOOKING GLASS

She is surely dead by now.

The nurse who settled her into the examining room, took her temperature, pulse, and blood pressure, and then asked her to strip down to her underwear, described Margaret in the chart with a single sentence: "58-year-old with inflammatory breast cancer here for surgical evaluation." The nurse might have also written that Margaret was the married mother of two grown children, had a successful accounting practice, and was on the verge of dying from a late case of the most aggressive kind of breast cancer.

Instead, she handed me the chart, sighed, and said while walking away to get the next waiting patient, "Good luck. This is a tough one."

I walked into the room where Margaret sat on an examining table, a flimsy polyester-blend hospital gown covering her chest. Her short brown hair formed a coiffed halo, and when she smiled, the outer corners of her blue eyes turned slightly downward rather than up. She looked like a well-worn Statue of Liberty.

Almost a year earlier, while taking a shower, Margaret had noticed a lump in her right breast. She thought that her breasts were lumpy to begin with, so she paid little attention. Several months later, she developed an open sore over the lump, but she thought it might have been because of an ill-fitting brassiere.

"Did the lump grow at all?" I asked.

"Yeah, I guess so," she replied. Her voice was flat, embellished with only a nasal drawl. She looked at me for a moment, blue eyes dull, then continued, "But I thought it was just swelling. You know, my breast lumps do change all the time."

I nodded and then asked her when she first decided to see a doctor.

"When my husband noticed a smell," she replied, her eyes never wavering from mine.

There was a faint odor: obviously human, but overripe and fleshy, like raw meat left out in the heat for too long.

I smiled and moved forward to examine Margaret. I put my fingers on her head and throat first and then gently pulled away the left side of the hospital gown to look at her unaffected breast. The breast felt lumpy, but it was not out of the ordinary. I reached up into her left armpit to feel for lymph nodes; again, there was nothing remarkable.

I covered Margaret's left chest and then lifted up the gown's right side. The smell in the room suddenly intensified. Grossly misshapen, Margaret's right breast had several rocklike tumors pushing out from beneath the tightly drawn skin. Over the largest mass there was a half-dollar-sized ulcer. The tumor below had grown so rapidly it had eaten away at her skin and spit out dead tissue. Three smaller craters circled the largest one like satellites.

The rotting smell in the room filled my head. I stood frozen in front of my patient, unwilling to examine her chest yet unable to cover her again. Margaret seemed oblivious. But as I stood there gaping at her tumor, all I wanted to do was ask what in the world had taken her so long to seek help.

For years afterward, long after Margaret had probably died, I believed that I could never arrive at the same place she did: a woman so confident of her own immortality, she was unaware of the degradation of her own body. I was different from Margaret. If I discovered a lump in the shower one morning, I would not accept it as part of my normal breast geography. If that lump grew, I would not consider it mere swelling. And if my own mortality stared me down, I would be the first to acknowledge it—straight on, without hesitation, and without any blinders.

No matter how many times I went over Margaret's story in my head or subsequently encountered similar patients—denying growing cancers, heart attacks, or AIDS—I viewed these patients as utterly foreign, living with a kind of distortion of reality that I wanted to believe bordered on the pathologic. After all, mortality was a part of my life and a part of my work; it was routine. And after nearly a decade of training, I believed that I had become very comfortable with death, even the idea of my own.

Like Ivan in Tolstoy's *The Death of Ivan Ilyich*, our own death is entirely irrational.

The syllogism he had learned from Kiesewetter's Logic—"Caius is a man, men are mortal, therefore Caius is mortal"—had always seemed to him correct as applied to Caius, but by no means to himself. That man Caius represented man in the abstract, and so the reasoning was perfectly sound; but he was not Caius, not an abstract man; he had always been a creature quite, quite distinct from all the others.

At times some of us openly test our convictions, engaging in hobbies, jobs, and activities that are in defiance of our essential humanness. As a resident, I cared for a man in his early thirties who was devoted to riding his motorcycle fast, helmet-free, and without concern for the usual legal limitations. On his third visit to our emergency room, with his most severe injuries yet—multiply fractured femur, pelvis, and ribs—I asked him if he had ever considered finding another hobby. He began laughing so hard that I thought the gurney would collapse beneath his quivering hairy belly. He told me between laughs that he planned to hop right back on his bike as soon as we discharged him.

Oddly, while we have difficulty accepting the inevitability of our own or our loved one's death, we can acknowledge a complete stranger's death with ease. For these unknown persons, we possess a cold rationality unavailable to ourselves. We comprehend the finality of death and the consequences of death-defying behavior, and in some instances we even use this understanding for our own benefit, taking the certitude of another's end to empower ourselves. Writing on the eve of World War I, Freud observed that during war, these strangers' deaths served not only political but also psychological ends; in witnessing others dying, we made ourselves survivors, and that survival reinforced our own sense of immortality.

It comes as no surprise, then, that physicians have a heightened sense of immortality.

On average, a physician in training sees twenty-eight deaths per year, or one death roughly every two weeks. Multiplied by the three to five or more years required for clinical training, that number would by force seem to make death frighteningly routine. "Surviving" the illnesses and deaths of others creates the kind of illusory immortality that leads not only to professional arrogance but also to those selfless feats of medical heroism.

I never kept count of all the patients I saw die. But I do remember the year when I saw the most death; it was also the year I saved the most lives. And in the midst of all those saves, my view of those who died changed. I forgot their humanity. I forgot that they had families and friends, likes and dislikes, and hopes probably not that dissimilar from my own. For me, these dead were just another middle-of-the-night operation.

During that year, the first year of my transplant fellowship, I performed almost a hundred procurements on brain-dead donors. I was part of a three-person traveling surgical team; and in the darkness of night, we rode in small jets, helicopters, limousines, and unmarked vans to far-flung hospitals on the West Coast. We dragged our empty coolers into strange hospitals, ignoring the odd stares from hospital personnel and wandering, insomniac patients. We maneuvered through the hospital's bowels, through corridors, basements, and elevators, finally finding our way to the operating room enclaves.

The work was like what we did in almost every other operation; we used the same instruments, techniques, and precautions. There were patients who, because of their anatomic anomalies, obesity, or scarring from multiple previous operations, made the operation more difficult;

and there were others whose bodies seemed made for a surgeon's hands.

After scrubbing in quiet meditation, we entered the familiar sanctity of the OR and approached the table. The donor, declared brain-dead hours earlier by the hospital's doctors, lay waiting for us, still connected to life support machinery. In a series of well-orchestrated and deliberate steps, we began our work upon the legally dead, keeping the body physiologically functioning until we had completed the initial dissection.

Once traversed by the scalpel, the skin of these dead bled with a ferocity that seemed unmistakably alive. Their chests rose and fell so regularly that I no longer saw the ventilator at the head of the bed. These patients' intestines, ignorant of death, slithered and pushed along half-digested boluses of food within their silky lumens.

Finally, when we were all but ready to lift the organs away from the body, we disconnected the machines. The shorter the time we exposed the organs to the stillness of death—noncirculating blood and the very early stages of decay—the better chances of success in the waiting recipients. The senior surgeon would place his steel clamp around the patient's aorta, and I would tug down on the diaphragm to expose the vena cava's entrance into the heart. With a bellow deep from my core I would yell, "Cross-clamp!" The anesthesiologists would disconnect the breathing tube, the senior surgeon would ratchet closed the aorta, and I would snip across the vena cava, letting the blood enter the suction tubes that filled clear wastebasket-sized canisters on the floor until the heart, first writhing and then skipping, would finally fall still.

The senior surgeon who accompanied me on most of those procurements that first year was Hasan, a man who had probably performed more of these operations than anyone in the United States. His goal was to extricate meticulously but rapidly each organ while leaving the body as intact as possible out of respect for the patient and family. Over and over again, he led me through the steps until our operations became an exquisitely choreographed ballet.

To Hasan, despite the legal status of the patient on the table, these harvests were a serious art form and a kind of spiritual mission. For me, these operations changed the balance of my world. I was spectator to the final passing of all of these nearly one hundred patients that year, but I would emerge from the operating rooms feeling more alive than when I had entered. I was energized by the act of operating, the hope of transplantation, and perhaps by my brush with death yet again.

By the time I had harvested from fifteen brain-dead donors, I could perform the operation not as an assistant but as the primary surgeon. By the time I had procured from thirty, I could lead a more inexperienced surgeon through each step. By patient number forty-five, I felt I could do the operation in my sleep or with one hand tied behind my back.

And by the time I had operated on more than sixty donors, my own immortality was beyond question.

My eighty-third organ procurement patient had a youthful body. I guess I paid more attention than usual because she, like me, was a thirty-five-year-old Asian American woman, and I had not operated on many. Her warm yellow skin was still taut, with few blemishes or folds; and reclining as she was, she could have been mistaken from a distance for any of the women lying on Santa Monica's beaches on Saturday afternoons.

On closer view, however, I could see that the flare of her hips and thighs had the deepening sweeps of a metabolism beginning to slow, and the skin on her fingertips and knuckles was thickened though still wrapped snugly around the muscles and bones. Her breasts were smallish, and her belly, which expanded slightly with each inspiration, was soft and hung between her two pelvic bones like an island hammock drawn tightly. Three white thunderbolts of stretched skin zigzagged down her pelvis, but the skin on her legs was smooth, the shins shiny. Her feet were meticulously pedicured. The skin that encircled each pedal digit was dewy, and her toenails, painted and filed, looked as if they had been dipped in pink spun sugar.

Three days earlier she had been driving with her ten-year-old son on a small southern California road when a drunk driver collided into her car at fifty miles per hour. Her son had died at the scene, but she was still alive, albeit with withering vital signs. As the paramedics extricated her body from the manacles of the car turned steel trap, they saw her grimacing, lips stretched back and jaw clamped so tightly that the rim of her mandible looked as if it would burst through the skin. She clenched her fists, extending her arms and legs relentlessly as the paramedics slid her into their ambulance. The paramedics recognized these tortured movements: the last repetitive and nonsensical neural signals of a dying brain.

In the trauma bay of the local hospital, the physicians and nurses resuscitated her with an array of machines and an assortment of intravenous medications. With large blunt-nosed shears, the nurses snipped off all her clothing, exposing her still-warm skin to the cool fluorescent glow of the room. They slipped off her wedding ring and gold necklace and put them in a small plastic bag that they taped to her medical chart. The intern silently and efficiently completed his triad of duties: drew an arterial blood sample, performed a rectal exam, and slid a catheter into her bladder. The head doctor barked orders, commanding silence in the hopelessly chaotic room and calling in more and more specialists.

By the time they had done all the tests and all the scans and cleaned off the blood and ground-in dirt and broken glass and changed the bloody sheets, the woman looked as if she had simply fallen asleep on the small trauma stretcher. Her eyes were closed, her breathing seemed peacefully regular, and her dark hair fell neatly over the sides of the gurney. Except for the plastic tubes, monitors, and wheezing ventilator machine that surrounded her, she might have even been mistaken for a tired surgeon who had sneaked off for a moment to rest in that quiet corner of the emergency room.

I looked up to the head of the operating table at the woman's face. A clear breathing tube snaked into her mouth, drops of moisture condensing within the plastic lumen. I saw her bruised lip and a black-and-blue eyelid that was swollen closed. A few strands of black hair strayed from underneath a dark towel wrapped around her head, like weeds that had grown insistently through the cracks of a sidewalk.

Hasan was working down in the abdomen. He wanted to open it quickly to assess the condition of the woman's liver. I needed to expose the heart and inferior vena cava.

I placed the tip of the Bovie, a pencil-like electrocautery instrument, into the small divot at the top of the donor's breastbone. As I moved my arm to begin the incision, the sterile drape covering her right breast fell away slightly. I pulled it up again to cover all except the area of the incision but noticed the undulations of each rib to the left of her breast and the very gentle fall of the breast tissue to her side. Her nipple and areola peeked through; they had a coloring and shape that I had only ever seen on one other person: myself. In fact, the very shape of her breast, the thinness of her chest, and the texture of her skin reminded me of my own upper body. It was as if I were standing naked after a shower, looking in a mirror.

I stopped for a moment, unable to put my instrument back to her breastbone. Hasan had already begun his portion of the operation, and I could smell the flesh burnt by the path of his cauterizing pen. It was a familiar scent—surgeons use the Bovie in almost every operation they do—but this time it felt as if the smell had found its way into the pit of my stomach. I stepped back from the table for a moment, tasting the smell in my mouth, and looked away to try to breathe in anything but what was wafting up into the air.

Hasan looked up from his work. "Are you sleepy?" he asked gently. The clock read 3:00 a.m.

I looked at the patient's chest. "No. I'm all right," I replied, trying to recover. "Just a little spacey."

Hasan motioned for me to move down to the patient's belly and stand across from him. "Come here a minute and feel her liver," he said. "It's perfect." He took my hand and plunged it into the woman's upper abdomen. The edges of the abdominal incision closed around my forearm, and it looked as if her body were swallowing me. My fingers felt lost in the warm sponginess of organs, loops of bowel sliding by, and her pulsating aorta gently and rhythmically nudging my palm. Her liver did feel perfect—soft, smooth, with sharp, well-formed edges.

Hasan told me he wanted to see the liver. Her insides made a gentle sloshing sound as I drew my hand out of her belly. I tried to pull open her incision, but her skin and abdominal wall had a vibrant elasticity that resisted my retraction. I looked closer at the cut edge and noticed that her dermis, the layer between the fat and the outer skin, was particularly thick. It was glossy white, free of any muscles, and shiny and strong from the myriad molecular cross-linkings of collagen.

As an intern in what I thought was the ultimate sacrifice to pedagogy, I had let several medical students place intravenous peripheral catheters in my arms for practice. Without fail, they always commented on my skin; driving those big needles through it and into the vein lying directly underneath was always difficult. "Thick skin," I would say, trying to make a dopey joke about the difficulties of internship. But then in all seriousness I would add, "My dermis is probably pretty thick." Looking at this woman's dermis now, I became acutely aware again of needles being driven into my arms and of the small swath of skin on my belly that was leaning against the operating table and touching her covered arm. That arm was warm, and through the layers of gowns and drapes, I felt the irregularities that were her fingers.

For a moment I saw a reflection of my own life and I felt as if I were pulling apart my own flesh. As we snipped away at the organ attachments, preparing to take her liver, pancreas, and kidneys, I wanted to ignore the aliveness of her body, to realize that she was in fact only a cadaveric reflection of myself. But then I could not bear to think of herself—myself—as dead and would once again think in my confused, sleep-deprived state of her as alive. The drape across her chest continued to slip, and I would have to see her breast yet again and then cover it. Her thick dermis seemed to buck constantly against our attempts to keep her belly open, making it difficult to keep my eyes off that strong, thick layer of tissue below the skin.

In the end, when we closed her stone-cold body, her

warm blood replaced by icy preservation solution, my mind felt as emptied as her abdominal cavity. The muscles in my palms ached, and my legs were numb. I was profoundly exhausted, from sleep deprivation, overwork, and an unbearable, unspeakable grief.

Soon after that procurement, I began to write stories. Not much, for when faced with a decision between eating and sleeping for the first time in seventy-two hours or writing, the primal needs won out every time. But when I finished my training a year later, fortified with the relatively regular meals and sleep of an attending surgeon, I began to write with some consistency. To my surprise, the writing seemed to pour out from a locked-up data bank within, oftentimes in unmitigated, logorrheic, and exhausting bursts. And the fictional stories I thought I was creating were almost always thinly veiled narratives about my patients, many of whom had passed away sometime in the last decade.

I enrolled in a couple of writing courses, with the hope that a class would help harness some of these impulses. Halfway through one course, the teacher asked to meet with me. I expected that she would want to discuss my repeating the course, since I had missed so many classes because of transplants. Or that she might want to discuss toning down the graphic clinical details. Instead all she said was: "Pauline, you *have* to write these stories."

I began to write the truth, painfully uncovering each fictional persona and finding the memory within. It was as if my teacher's words had liberated me to do what I wanted to do. I tossed the memories around, each time excavating a detail that would come alive again with excruciating clarity. I collected the pieces, first in bound notebooks and then, when that became too cumbersome, in the hard drive of my computer. And when I read through them again, I wept with both unresolved grief and a deep sense of shame.

That is when I began to see what I had become.

I once attended a lecture given by a nationally prominent surgeon, known famously for his experience in a set of particularly difficult operations and infamously for his own countless submissions to the plastic surgeon's knife. Although he easily could have been my grandfather, his face was wrinkle-free, his skin like plastic wrap stretched tightly over a bowl. Every so often during his one-hour talk, he would break into a huge grin that, to my amazement, would miraculously leave his flawless skin undisturbed.

I had never seen the medical school auditorium so crowded. The man was a legend in medicine, having revolutionized surgery and cured thousands of patients. He was probably the childhood hero of every surgeon in that audience, including me. In addition to his well-known fearless appetite for the greatest of surgical challenges, the speaker had managed to cultivate a kind of swashbuckling public image so that his personal and professional lives competed for greater notoriety. I wanted as much to catch a glimpse of him as to hear what he had to present.

To the audience's delight, the surgeon's lecture was not a serious, informative talk but a sort of historical show-and-tell, relaying the details of his training and the highlights of his career. On the screen he flashed pictures from his youth; he had trained with some of the great legends of medicine and surgery. There were multiple photos of his patients both young and old, with decrepit "before" and robust, smiling "after" pictures. Finally, he came to a photo of his surgical team. The speaker sat in the center of the photo, sterile mask hanging casually at his neck and surgical cap jauntily askew. About a half dozen other surgeons, similarly dressed, surrounded him. On his lap the speaker held a large sign that read simply *100,000*.

At this point the speaker stopped talking, looked up at the audience, and flashed that improbable grin. There was a series of gasps and reverent "ah"s from the audience. I heard one surgeon, famous at our institution for his own technical wizardry, whisper loudly, "Damn!" with a mix of awe and envy. The picture, the speaker began to explain after the murmurs had finally died down, was taken after he had performed the one hundred thousandth such surgical case, clearly establishing him as the leader in experience in these kinds of procedures.

That afternoon the conversations in most of the operating rooms centered on the morning's lecture. A friend who was also an anesthesia colleague listened quietly as the surgical residents and I discussed the speaker's talk. She rolled her eyes as she heard us recount what he had said, and one half of her mouth curled up in disdain. She finally interrupted us and said, "That man just fears death, doesn't he?"

Medicine is replete with stories of those like that morning's lecturer who will go to superhuman lengths to cure their patients. These doctors become the highly respected heroes of physicians everywhere, and while not all of us choose to make similar personal sacrifices, these legends set the professional bar to which we all aspire. In a way, they become the attendings for the profession as a whole.

In the confines of our hospitals and our own particular practices, we imitate these fearless efforts to cure. During my training I watched my attendings—seemingly immune to fatigue and hunger—stitching, removing stitches, then putting them back in and pushing onward in an attempt to save their patients in the operating room. I remember one particular case from my internship. After not eating, drinking, or sleeping for forty-eight hours, I was seeing stars in every corner of the warm OR, and my head felt like a lead weight that could tip over any minute and pull the rest of me down to the floor or right into the patient's opened body. My attending surgeon was oblivious to any concept of personal discomfort, let alone the discomfort of some intern struggling to hold the patient's liver out of the operating field and stay awake. Over the course of the next few hours he worked obsessively, calling in more and more residents and staff to help with this bloody and eventually doomed patient.

Just as easily, however, we physicians can slip from the dramatic heroics into a well-worn pattern of denial. Denial, after all, is a way of coping that we learn early and well as first-year medical students, suppressing our anxieties as we carve away at the cadaveric remains of fellow human beings. Over time we come to believe so deeply that sublimating our fear of death makes us better doctors that some of us will skip around the very word during our conversations with terminal patients. We will work almost maniacally to forestall the inevitable but then stubbornly, when death becomes inescapable, refuse to face it for fear of losing our focus on the goal of cure.

All of this is not to say that such endeavors are futile or that physicians are fundamentally incapable of changing in order to provide better care for patients. The psychological roots of our behavior are profound; still, we entered this field to help other people, whether that means curing their diseases or helping them die gracefully.

Spurred on by more aggressive patient advocacy and by a paradoxical insight into our own fallibility, we have begun changing the way our profession teaches and approaches care of the dying.

Research, for example, has been flourishing. The Open Society Institute's Project on Death in America gave away $45 million over nine years for work devoted to palliative and end-of-life care; and researchers continue to find funding support through the National Institutes of Health and the Robert Wood Johnson Foundation. In 1985 the *Journal of Palliative Care* was launched, and in 1998 the American Academy of Hospice and Palliative Medicine (AAHPM) started the *Journal of Palliative Medicine* in order to accommodate the growing interest in palliative care. AAHPM itself has grown from 250 founding members in 1988 to more than 2,000 members in early 2005.

Educational opportunities have increased as well. The number of medical schools offering occasional lectures or elective courses on death and dying increased to 97 percent in 1998. That number should soon reach 100 percent; the Liaison Committee on Medical Education, the national accrediting authority for medical schools, now requires that all U.S. and Canadian medical schools include end-of-life care in their curricula.

There have also been significant changes in training. The American Board of Internal Medicine recently began requiring residents to participate in some curriculum training on palliative care; and the American College of Surgeons has begun developing pilot palliative care programs for surgical residents. Moreover, twenty subspecialty fellowships nationwide are in palliative care. In June 2006, the American Council of Graduate Medical Education decided to accredit these fellowship programs; three months later, the American Board of Medical Specialities voted to confer official subspecialty status and offer certification in Hospice and Palliative Medicine.

Even the training grounds for young doctors—the academic medical centers—have begun to change. In a recent survey of one hundred academic medical centers, more than a quarter offered some form of palliative care consultation or an inpatient palliative care unit; an additional 20 percent of centers were planning to add such programs in the near future. This growth parallels the increase in all hospitals; the percentage of U.S. hospitals with such programs went from 15 percent in 2001 to 25 percent in 2003.

A psychiatrist friend once said to me, "We are in the business of suffering." Most of us are drawn to medicine because we want to ease that suffering, but we forget over time that it encompasses more than just diseases and their symptoms.

What is more significant for our patients, particularly those at the end of life, is the suffering which results from a loss of meaning and purpose. This suffering is profound, but it is *not* hopeless. We physicians can address it by being present for our patients, by giving weight to their experience, and by becoming the kind of doctors we have always wanted to be.

But first we must be able to acknowledge our own mortality. Given the scope of the recent reforms, it seems that this acknowledgment has begun.

About two years ago I received a follow-up telephone call from the brother-in-law of a former patient. My patient, Alfred, had founded a successful chain of ice cream stores in southern California. When he reached sixty-five, he developed cholangiocarcinoma. Though jaundiced, he still retained his handsome features: thick salt-and-pepper hair, a Roman nose, and high dramatic cheekbones. Alfred wanted a second opinion about the feasibility of a curative operation and came to our clinic. By the time I saw him, his tumor had spread beyond his liver, and we could do little surgically. Instead, we placed a tube in his bile ducts to bypass the tumor and help drain his bile.

During his short stay with us, I visited him every day to make sure that his jaundice was resolving and that he was learning how to deal with the new tube poking out of the right side of his abdomen. Alfred was not a naturally warm man; it took a fair number of visits before he was at ease with me. One afternoon he told me about a dream he had had. In this dream he was lying in a coffin-like box made of brick. As he lay there unable to move, he saw a faceless group of people placing layer after layer of bricks around him so that eventually he was almost entirely sealed within the brick box. He wanted to run, but his legs would not budge. He wanted to breathe, but he could not get any air. He wanted to scream, but no voice would come forth.

"I'm going to try chemotherapy," he said to me afterward. We had discussed the poor responses to chemotherapy that characterize cholangiocarcinoma. "When the time comes, I want to be at home and be comfortable and be with my family," Alfred said, "but right now, I don't want to be passive in my box." He smiled. "Besides, someone has got to run my business, and my kid isn't about to do it from New Guinea." Alfred and his wife, Judy, were fond of talking about their three children, particularly their son, who had become an anthropologist and was unreachable, doing fieldwork in a far corner of the world. Alfred made an appointment with a medical oncologist who worked in a different hospital and who had been recommended by a friend of his.

Six months later Judy brought Alfred back to us when he became confused at home. His liver was failing, allowing the waste products of metabolism to accumulate to toxic levels. Without a functioning liver or aggressive medical therapy, he would slip into a coma within a day or so and would die soon thereafter. Judy was distraught. Her husband had become slightly confused a week earlier, but the medical oncologist had said they would hold off on chemo for a day or two and that Alfred would be fine. He had never talked about Alfred's liver failing or about the possibility that he might die. When Alfred became confused again, the doctor told Judy to send her husband to our hospital, not his own; he would see Alfred in his office after discharge for another round of chemotherapy.

Alfred had changed dramatically. His lush hair had thinned to a few wispy strands. Fluid had accumulated in his belly and had blown his torso up so tightly that his skin was almost transparent. His face was so wasted that his tongue appeared bloated, the rough surface coated with a layer of desiccated medications. His lips were dry and peeling like the paint of an old house. The jaundice, which had begun to resolve by the end of his initial stay with us, had vividly returned.

Looking at Alfred, I knew that we could transfer him into the intensive care unit; put tubes into his mouth, nose, bladder, and rectum; hook him up to a ventilator; and probably cure his confusion. But he was dying and any remedy would be temporary. When I mentioned all the possible options to Judy, she began to cry. "I know what Alfred wants," she said. "I just can't believe this is coming now."

Alfred appeared to be sleeping, unaware of my conversation with his wife. His breath made a rumbling sound as it coursed through his throat, but every few minutes he would speak nonsensically in an unfamiliar high-pitched voice, only to lapse back to the low-pitched rumbles. As I went to kneel at the side of his bed, I remembered our earlier conversation about his dream. I bent over so my face was close to his. His wife came over as well, crying silently and wiping her nose with a limp and ragged tissue. "Mr. Lipstein," I said to Alfred. His eyes remained closed and his breathing heavy and uneven. "We can either take you to the intensive care unit or we can let you go home. I'm not sure how much longer we have, but I want to know what you want." Although I asked Alfred, I was almost certain that he was too somnolent to respond.

His lids opened for a minute and his dark eyes focused on mine. I was startled by the sudden clarity in his gaze; it was as if the Alfred I had seen six months earlier had returned. "Dr. Chen," he said in a deep voice that was both resonant and lucid. "Let me go home." He closed his eyes and lapsed back into his semiconscious state.

That morning I called hospice and we arranged to send Alfred home.

A few days after Alfred's funeral, his brother-in-law called to thank me for helping Alfred die at home. The people from hospice had been "like angels" and supported not only Alfred but also his wife and family. Judy Lipstein was upset that their medical oncologist had done nothing earlier to prevent the last trip to the hospital, a trip she believed really "took it out of him," but she was grateful to have had her husband at home at the end. He was comfortable, peaceful in his own room, and even alert for part of a day.

He died a week after he left the hospital. The evening that he died, he slipped into a coma and his breathing became irregular, halting for a minute and then resuming with a startle. He began wailing, a low, soft cry with each breath. The hospice nurses told Judy that they had seen this before; it was the cry of the dying, the death rattle, the last sighs, a final goodbye to the living. In the end all of Alfred's family came home, even the anthropologist son, whom they had managed to contact soon after Alfred left our hospital. Holding Alfred and one another, they surrounded him during his last moments.

I closed my eyes as Alfred's brother-in-law recounted those last moments, because I had seen it before. This time, however, the face of the dying person in my mind was Alfred's. The pauses in Alfred's breathing grew longer, the wailing stopped, and the expression on his face became more serene until there was only stillness.

The brother-in-law's voice cracked on the other end of the line, and I felt that same wave of helplessness from deep in my chest. I wondered silently why I still could not save my patient despite all the knowledge and training and technology. I began to speak, saying what I always did with grieving loved ones. I wish I could have cured him, I wish I could have done more.

But then I heard Alfred's brother-in-law thanking me yet again for helping Alfred die at home and with his family. "You know, Dr. Chen," he said, "it was just as he had wished."

It was then I realized that I *had* done more. I had comforted my patient and his family. I had eased their suffering. I had been present for them during life and despite death.

I had caught a glimpse of the doctor I could become.

EPILOGUE

Thirty minutes after I sent the first draft of this book to my editor, an e-mail with the subject line "Query on liver, oncologists" popped up in my in-box. It was from Dorinne, one of my college anthropology professors.

These sorts of e-mails come to me fairly frequently. I like my profession, and there is a kind of semi-illicit pleasure in doling out medical opinions for free and without requiring my "patients" to wait. Of all the friends and family members I help, few give me more satisfaction than my former teachers.

I first heard about Dorinne over Sunday brunch. My college friends and I, convinced we were practicing important conversational skills, had elevated mealtime socializing—and procrastination—to new heights. The *ne plus ultra* of these mealtime discussions were Sunday brunches, when our conversations would last far beyond the 2:00 p.m. closing time and well into the 5:00 p.m. early dinners of the more dedicated students in our ranks. Sometimes these conversations focused on politics, other times they wandered to the couplings of our friends. One

Sunday afternoon early in my sophomore year, a friend began talking about Dorinne.

"Pauline," she said. "You have *got* to go to one of Dorinne's lectures. She's amazing. She'll change the way you think. And," my friend lowered her voice to a whisper, "she is *so* cool."

My friend's comments were serious recommendations on a campus where Nobel laureates flourished and the weight of the college course catalogue rivaled that of my science textbooks. I looked up Dorinne's lecture schedule and went to her next talk.

I was one of those college students whose mind had the terrible propensity to wander during lectures. But for that one hour, I could barely pull my focus away from Dorinne long enough to take notes. She pulled out theory after accepted theory in her field, unraveled them by nonchalantly tugging on the stray ends, and then replaced them with ideas so skillfully woven that the old paradigms instantly became obsolete. And even among the diverse population that inhabited my college world, Dorinne stood out. She was one of less than a handful of Asian American professors in my college, wore black, sported an asymmetrical haircut, and, at the end of her talk, trotted away from the lectern in heels that bordered on stiletto.

Over the course of four years I took as many courses as I could from Dorinne. One year I invited her to a faculty-student dinner at my dormitory. Would this brilliant professor, I wondered as I welcomed her to our dining hall, be comfortable eating our college student grub? As we talked over dinner, I learned that her life was as odd a mix of Asian and American as mine and that she talked as easily about parents, clothing, and food as she did about politics and hermeneutics. And often she intertwined the topics in the most mind-bending of ways.

She brought up one of her current projects that she thought I might find interesting given our conversation. "I'm looking at how Asian Americans are portrayed in fashion and theater," she said, pushing her fork into the evening's meal of chicken, mashed potatoes, and misshapen olive-green peas. "Specifically, I am trying to examine how myths about race, gender, and nationality shape the Asian American experience."

I could barely respond. All those hours practicing witty, scintillating conversation in the dining halls had been for naught.

In the midst of that existential angst which is young adulthood, Dorinne became my mentor, big sister, friend, and rock star all rolled into one. She was living proof that despite the worried counsel of my parents and the challenges of my peers, I could reach for all that I wanted to be. And after she took to calling me one of her "women warriors," everything became possible.

After I graduated I saw Dorinne once but then lost touch until I finished my surgical training. Over the last few years we have e-mailed occasionally. She is now a full professor in a well-respected anthropology department, author of two critically acclaimed books, and an award-winning playwright. I am the former student who became a surgeon. And although her work is as far from operating as one could get, I still find myself drawn to Dorinne's writing. I will pull her books out from time to time and imagine myself in that lecture hall once again. I will hear her voice, pulling at the loose threads of my mind, unraveling and then reworking them until the fabric that connects my thoughts seems stronger than ever. And then in the next paragraph she will begin that unraveling again, as if her job as my mentor will never be done.

. . .

Dorinne's e-mail began with an apology. "Thank you so much for your Christmas card, and I'm sorry I've been so poor a correspondent." She had been feeling under the weather for a month and finally went to see a doctor who ordered several tests.

"It turns out that I have 'suspicious-looking' nodules on my liver," began the second paragraph. I re-read the words; they did not make sense. I fiddled with my computer, as if it had somehow mangled the message it was transmitting.

"It turns out that I have 'suspicious-looking' nodules on my liver." I stopped breathing for a minute; my head felt at first so light I had to hold my seat, and then so full I thought it would burst. I kept reading. "I go in today for blood work and an ultrasound," she continued. "The doctor thinks it looks like liver cancer."

By the time I finished reading the e-mail, I felt that familiar pressure in my head; by evening, it had blossomed into a headache so severe that the Tylenol in my bathroom cabinet could not quell it. I spent that night making arrangements for Dorinne to see the best specialists in her city. I described her case to the other doctors, but my mind kept fast-forwarding to the future. I tried to stop my racing thoughts, but there was no button to push and nowhere else to look. I saw the tumor devouring her liver, then spitting out voracious offspring that would eat away at her intestines and lungs. I saw the rocky cancer oozing the malignant fluid that would cause her belly to swell. I saw an end that I knew I could not prevent.

And I was left wondering as I began that free fall of grief yet again: what had really changed?

.   .   .

We cannot remove the pain of loss. Death—whether of patients or of loved ones—will always be difficult. We can create reforms, we can institute policy changes, and we can even write books. But our professional fear and aversion to dying is the most difficult—and most fundamentally human—obstacle in changing end-of-life care. Our grief is the price we pay for caring for the terminally ill, and our aversion is the weight that anchors our inertia and denial.

Through the many phone calls and e-mails in which I would try to help Dorinne, I realized that all those reform efforts could not mitigate my grief. What they did do, however, was break my free fall. Those new standards of care for patients at the end of life were the guideposts I could lean upon even though my vision was clouded by despair. The policy changes of my profession encouraged me to discuss even when my natural response was to deny and ignore. And finally, the act of writing this book gave me insight into my own anxiety: its roots, its persistence, and its crippling presence. In the end, acknowledging mortality—both Dorinne's and my own—liberated me; it allowed me to be present for my beloved college mentor.

Ten excruciating days later, the results of much additional testing revealed that the mass in Dorinne's liver was a rare benign tumor. She wrote me:

I can't thank you enough; you've been instrumental in helping me get back my life. If anything, this has taught me how precious friends are. Thank you for the inexpressibly touching and life-giving gift of your friendship. It's wonderful to have friends who, as they say in Japanese, "do me the honor of worrying about me."

That honor of worrying—of caring, of easing suffering, of being present—may be our most important task, not only as friends but as physicians, too.

And when we are finally capable of that, we will have become true healers.

ACKNOWLEDGMENTS

It would require another chapter to list all those who have supported me in writing this book, but there are several individuals who deserve special mention.

There are two people to whom I am particularly indebted and without whom this book would have never come about: my agent, Rebecca Gradinger, and my editor, Jordan Pavlin. Both supported me unfailingly, even as the work overlapped with their respective pregnancies and what became—on my account—*working* maternity leaves. From the very beginning, Rebecca stood by me with her friendship, uncanny intuition, sense of humor, honesty, and perfectly timed words of inspiration. Jordan, with her brilliant editorial skills, insight, warmth, and generous encouragement, lovingly shepherded this manuscript to a level far beyond what I ever believed I was capable of producing. I cannot thank Rebecca and Jordan enough for believing in me and in this book.

I am profoundly indebted to my patients. All of them, not only those on these pages, and their families gave me far more than I ever gave them. I hope this book has done some justice to their grace, courage, and generosity.

Three other individuals have been particularly important: Daniel Minton, without whom I would have never closed my eyes and jumped; Shauna Sorensen, whose confidence in me never for a moment wavered; and Ronald W. Busuttil, who has been my surgical father *always.*

Early on and in particularly meaningful ways, Peter Ginna, Ted Genoways and *The Virginia Quarterly Review,* Holiday Reinhorn, Gary Glickman, Russell Martin, and Lydia Nibley all supported me in my writing endeavors.

I am deeply indebted to Robert Burt and my dearest friend, Celia Chao, both of whom read through early drafts of the entire manuscript. While I take full responsibility for any errors or flaws, their astute insight and invaluable commentary strengthened this book immeasurably.

I am grateful to the academic mentors, colleagues, nurses, and health care professionals who have taught and supported me over the years, especially Myron Tong, the late Charles McKhann, Dorinne Kondo, Arthur Kleinman, John Baldwin, Rafael Amado, Sue McDiarmid, Hasan Yersiz, Jon Hiatt, Anne Sbarge, the late Morse Hamilton, Barbara Kosty, James Rugen, and Marcia and Edward Ward. Thank you, all.

No first-time author could be more fortunate than to land in the capable hands of the people at Knopf. Their meticulous attention to detail, thoughtfulness, and care rival that of the best surgeons I have ever worked with. I am deeply grateful to Sonny Mehta, Pat Johnson, Paul Bogaards, Christine Gillespie, Nicholas Latimer, Abby Weintraub, Maria Massey, Suzanne Smith, Soonyoung Kwon, and Thomas Dobrowolski. I have also had the great fortune of working with Sarah Gelman and Victoria Gerken, both of whom have been tireless sources of support, friendship, and much appreciated humor, and with Leslie Levine, editorial assistant extraordinaire.

Throughout my life, I have been able to turn to friends;

the writing of this book has been no exception. There are a few to whom I am particularly indebted: Susan M. Lerner, Andra Jurist, Joan Goldwyn, Erika Schillinger, JoAnn Busuttil, Patricia Lee Cirone, Joan Longwell, Chuu Fong Lea, Jacquelynne Wyeth Simpson, Paula Phipps and the Little Wagon Early Education Center, George W. Cole Jr., Leah Nero Pittle, Johanna Salamandra, Lucy Artinian, William Simon, Carmen Chang, Katherine Halsey, James Yun, Shiobhan Weston, Grace Jeon, Ruth Saxe, Ellie Sachse, and Jane Salodof MacNeil.

I must thank, too, my wonderful family. In particular, my siblings, Lena, Michael, and now Grace; Uncle Chung and Irene; my grandmother, Hwa-tze Wang; the "Big Kids"—Comfort, Bronwen, Brooke, Phoebe, and now Kit; my parents-in-law, Anne and Mac; and la famiglia Cope—Greg, Comfort, Eliza, and Thomas.

My parents deserve special thanks. Despite their difficulties as immigrants, they gave me a world-class education and enough emotional and financial support to get through all those years relatively unscathed. From my mother, Mei Rong Chen, I learned about insight and the power of determination; from my father, Jong Ping Chen, I learned about storytelling and the magnificence of human grace. I remain indebted to them.

Perhaps most important, I need to thank my husband and my daughters. Throughout all of this, Woody, who never expected that his surgeon bride would also be a writer, has been unwavering in his support. He has created a loving space in our lives for whatever my work entails and has maintained his equanimity even when asked to read yet another draft of the same chapter in an hour for the tenth time. Despite it all, he has unhesitatingly encouraged me even when that has meant doing more work than any 50-50 partnership should entail.

Woody, Natalie, and Isabelle bore the brunt of harried

schedules, endless revisions, and deadlines; yet they continued to shower me with more affection and love than any one person deserves. They are the light of my life, and they inspire me to be the best I can be.

And it is to them, and to my parents, that I dedicate this book.

NOTES

Introduction

xiii *But in a society where more than 90 percent:* L. L. Emanuel et al., "Gaps in End-of-Life Care." Those with chronic illness at the end of life will generally follow one of three trajectories: a short period of obvious decline at the end (e.g., cancer); long-term disability punctuated by exacerbations and unpredictable timing of death (e.g., chronic organ system failure); and self-care deficits and a decline marked by slowly dwindling health (e.g., frailty, dementia). An increasing number of people are now falling into the last category, yet our current health care system is premised on rapid, sudden deaths occurring secondary to trauma, heart attacks, and infections. Lynn, "Care at the Close of Life."

xiii *charged with shepherding the terminally ill:* Donaldson and Field, "Measuring Quality of Care."

xiii *Most patients and their families:* In 1997 the American Medical Association public opinion survey revealed that almost three quarters of Americans expect their physician to be both confident and competent in providing care should they develop life-threatening illnesses. L. L. Emanuel et al., "Gaps in End-of-Life Care."

xv *"[I]n the unconscious every one of us":* Freud, *Civilisation, War and Death.*

xv   *a good death, however each person may define that:* What individuals define as a "good death" has changed through time. Aries, *Hour of Our Death.* Moreover, individual definitions are heavily influenced by cultural, psychosocial, and spiritual meanings, as well as by physical care. Steinhauser et al., "Factors Considered Important"; Steinhauser et al., "A Good Death"; Walter, "Good Death."

xv   *"We remember the old saying":* Freud, *Civilisation, War and Death.*

Chapter 1
RESURRECTIONIST

8   *it has until recently been the only focus of medical schools:* Bertman and Marks, "Humanities in Medical Education."

8   *While all premedical students fully expect:* Several writers have described the difficulties medical students encounter during gross anatomy dissection. Giegerich, a journalist, followed a medical school class through the entire course. Giegerich, *Body of Knowledge.* F. W. Hafferty studied the experience from a sociological perspective. Hafferty, *Into the Valley.* Several physicians have also written about their own experiences. Klass, *Not Entirely Benign Procedure;* Rothman, *White Coat;* Sharkey, *A Parting Gift.*

8   *It was as if such separation:* Others have also written about the impact that such detachment has on medical students' future practices. Dyer, "Reshaping Our Views"; Fox, *Sociology of Medicine;* Hafferty, *Into the Valley.*

17   *"[D]issection requires in its practitioners":* Richardson, *Death, Dissection and the Destitute.*

17   *soon enough they are dissecting:* Roach, in her humorous but eye-opening book, writes that working with cadavers requires that medical students objectify and erase some of their cadavers' humanity. Roach, *Stiff.*

17   *The use of black humor:* Sociologist F. W. Hafferty posits that the use of black humor provides medical students with the following: emotional distance from the basic content and normative messages in the cadaver stories, emotional distance from the dominant symbolic presence of the cadaver as a human being, and a sanctioned and alternative source of emotions in the anatomy lab. Hafferty, "Cadaver Stories"; Hafferty, *Into the Valley.*

17   *The medical urban legends:* Hafferty also writes that these cadaver stories form part of the oral tradition of medical culture and thus are

an important part of the emotional socialization and acculturation of the not yet professional medical students. They "provide storytellers and their audience with an opportunity to demonstrate an awareness of, and commitment to, the underlying norms and traditions of this new and highly desired (medical) culture." Hafferty, "Cadaver Stories."

17 *"At times, it felt as if death"*: Rothman, *White Coat.*

18 *Some students misinterpret their painful reactions:* Bertman and Marks, "Humanities in Medical Education."

18 *There are experts in medical education:* Ibid.

18 *For example, more schools are now holding memorial services:* Ibid.; Marks et al., "Human Anatomy." Several years after I had graduated, Northwestern University's Feinberg School of Medicine, my alma mater, offered an elective seminar called "Reflections on Gross Anatomy." In this course, students explored and expressed their reactions to gross anatomy through literature and writing. Reifler, "Narratives of Gross Anatomy."

19 *A German anatomy atlas:* The first three volumes of Pernkopf's four-volume *Topographische Anatomie des Menschen* (Topographic Human Anatomy) were published between 1937 and 1945, and several revised editions, including one in English, were subsequently issued. This atlas was the introduction to death in medicine for generations of medical students. Eduard Pernkopf was one of the most respected Austrian medical academics at a time when Germany and Austria reigned supreme in the world of medicine. Pernkopf became dean of the Medical Faculty of Vienna in 1938, serving until 1945, and he was rector of the University of Vienna from 1943 to 1945. Along with his academic positions, he was also a high-ranking Austrian National Socialist and a confirmed anti-Semite. In 1997 the University of Vienna commissioned an investigation into the origins of the bodies used in several of the anatomic illustrations. It is likely that some of the corpses or parts of them were from victims of wartime Nazi atrocities. While Pernkopf did not personally murder for the cadavers in his atlas, he was likely aware of their origins (personal communication with Howard M. Spiro, M.D.). Spiro, "Silence of Words."

21 *For much of their history, anatomists and physicians:* McDowell, "Corpus and the Hare"; Mims, *When We Die;* Richardson, *Death, Dissection and the Destitute;* Tward and Patterson, "Grave Robbing to Gifting."

24   *One child's father even discovered:* This anecdote is strikingly similar
      to the urban legends recounted in medical school anatomy labs.
      F. W. Hafferty has written about five recurrent types of cadaver
      stories. The first type has medical students carrying cadavers or
      cadaver parts outside the lab to shock nonmedical people. The sec-
      ond involves the manipulation of a cadaver's sexual organs. The
      third, which Hafferty refers to as "resurrection" stories, involve the
      cadavers becoming more lifelike because students dress them or
      move them in ways that make the cadavers seem alive. In the fourth
      type, the cadaver is a relative or friend of the dissector (or, as in the
      case of this historical anecdote and the one involving Senator John
      Scott Harrison, the cadaver is related to a lay observer). The fifth
      type portrays the cadaver as food or as a receptacle for food. Haf-
      ferty, "Cadaver Stories"; Hafferty, *Into the Valley.*

24   *Instead, they found the body of Senator Harrison:* Twad and Patter-
      son, "Grave Robbing to Gifting."

25   *by employees at a California medical school:* Ornstein and Zarembo,
      "UCLA Body Parts Scandal."

25   *by a dentist and funeral home director:* Childress, "Body Snatchers";
      Hays, "Four Indicted."

Chapter 2
INTO THE NEXUS

35   *none of this had I ever seen on the screen:* Media depictions have a
      significant impact on public perceptions of cardiopulmonary resus-
      citation. For example, CPR succeeds much more frequently on tele-
      vision than in reality and often results in full recovery. Patients and
      families, under the influence of such misrepresentations, may make
      decisions that result in prolonged suffering and harm. Diem and Tul-
      sky, "Resuscitation on Television."

45   *this act of creating a new moral paradigm:* Fox, *Sociology of Medi-
      cine;* Hafferty, *Into the Valley.* Several doctors have also written
      "insider accounts" of this professionalization process. Klass, *Not
      Entirely Benign Procedure;* Konner, *Becoming a Doctor;* Rothman,
      White Coat.

46   *but seeing patients die bothered me:* Rhodes-Kropf et al. recently
      examined the responses of medical students to death. They found
      that medical students had emotionally powerful reactions, even in
      the absence of a significant clinical relationship with the patient.

Moreover, because of lack of discussion or emotional reaction from others around them, students often inferred that avoidance and continuing with work were appropriate coping reactions. Rhodes-Kropf et al., "Medical Students' Reactions."

51 *But when I looked over at Bill to ask:* In a recent survey, only one of forty-seven medical residents reported having had formal training either in medical school or during residency on how to determine death. Ferris et al., "When the Patient Dies."

Chapter 3
SEE ONE, DO ONE

60 *Premedical students overwhelmingly believe:* Chuck, "Do Premedical Students Know."

60 *"of all the professions":* Nuland, *How We Die.*

60 *Attracted to medicine:* Others have referred to this heightened anxiety over death among medical students and physicians and to the use of denial as a coping mechanism. Dickinson and Tournier, "Decade Beyond"; Ellard, "Being a Doctor"; Gabbard, "Compulsiveness in the Normal Physician"; Rhodes-Kropf et al., "Medical Students' Reactions."

61 *"[the] power of attendings":* Bosk, *Forgive and Remember.*

61 *We look to our attending physicians for guidance:* Several studies on the effect of patient deaths on physicians have shown that younger physicians report higher levels of anxiety and feel more personally responsible than older, more experienced doctors. Jackson et al., "Powerful Patient Deaths"; Kane and Hogan, "Death Anxiety." Unfortunately, many of these younger clinicians also experience these deaths in isolation. Jackson et al., "Powerful Patient Deaths"; Sullivan et al., "Status of Medical Education." A substantial percentage of trainees do not discuss deaths with their attendings, and when they do, the education and the support they receive is inadequate. Redinbaugh et al., "Doctors' Emotional Reactions"; Schwartz et al., "Medical Residents' Perceptions." Most residents instead tend to rely on talking with their peers, the other residents. Redinbaugh et al., "Doctors' Emotional Reactions."

61 *we learn that many of them:* In a recent survey of medical students, residents, and attendings on attitudes and experiences related to end-of-life care, researchers noted a large discrepancy in refusal rates. While only 8 percent of students and 13 percent of residents

refused to answer the twenty-five-minute telephone survey, almost 50 percent of the faculty refused. Most medical faculty who refused said they were not interested in the study. Others said that they were too busy, did not participate in such surveys, would not participate without payment, or, despite assurances from the investigators that their work qualified them for participation, felt that end-of-life care had no place in their work. Sullivan et al., "Status of Medical Education." While the researchers did not interpret these discrepancies, it would appear that the attending physicians either did not place a lot of importance on end-of-life care or denied its relevance to their work despite the researchers' assurance that they were indeed eligible for the study.

61 *Even our textbooks:* Rabow et al., "End-of-Life Care Content."

61 *We end up sifting through our own experiences:* In their study of surgery residents, Rappaport and Witzke found that only 50 percent of senior residents reported ever discussing death and dying with their attending surgeons. Rappaport et al., "Surgical Residency." Rappaport and Witzke later surveyed third-year medical students and found that over a third of students on their internal medicine rotations had never discussed with an attending physician how to deal with a terminal patient. Rappaport and Witzke, "Clinical Years of Medical School."

70 *During the mid-1990s:* SUPPORT Principal Investigators, "SUPPORT study."

71 *A high percentage of these patients continued to complain:* A subsequent study by Weiss et al. of almost one thousand terminally ill patients challenged the perception that pain is undertreated in the dying. These researchers found that less than a third of patients with moderate to severe pain and less than a quarter of all terminal patients who received treatment in the past month want more analgesia. Most patients were willing to tolerate pain because other considerations, such as avoiding the side effects of opioids, were more important. Weiss et al., "Experience of Pain." Based on these results, some experts believe that pain is thus a poor indicator of quality of care. However, interpreted differently, these results may indicate that we not only inadequately treat the side effects but also fail to address concerns and misperceptions among patients regarding opioids.

71 *One may be that physicians cannot bear:* Physicians may fear that any discussion about death or dying will eliminate patients' hope and depress them; however, neglecting such discussions can also

lead to unnecessary suffering and pain. Quill, "Care at the Close of Life."

71 *since dying patients are often under the care of myriad specialists:* Quill, "Care at the Close of Life."

72 *physicians will continue aggressive care because they fear litigation:* Hendricks, "Patients, Kin Want More." In their paper, Meisel et al. review the myths and realities of seven perceived legal barriers to end-of-life care, including the legal repercussions of using narcotic pain medications. Meisel et al., "Seven Legal Barriers." These fears are not unwarranted. In 1999, for example, Dr. Frank Fisher of Shasta County, California, was arrested and charged with drug trafficking and murder after aggressively treating his patients' pain with narcotics. After losing his home and practice and spending five months in jail, he was finally exonerated when it was discovered that the patients had died in accidents or from their medical illnesses. Satel, "Doctors Behind Bars."

72 *A significant number of patients also deny life-threatening illnesses:* S. D. Block, "Perspectives on Care."

72 *as many as 10 percent of patients hospitalized:* Chochinov et al., "Prognostic Awareness."

72 *Despite the researchers' efforts:* Burt, in his book *Death Is That Man Taking Names,* offers the most compelling explanation of these findings. "[D]eath has a more palpable presence in the enterprise of medicine than in most other endeavors and . . . the presence of death always conveys some sense of evil and injustice." Burt asserts that the SUPPORT physicians were not purposely causing suffering; instead, they were imposing a sense of order on a clinical world rendered chaotic by the presence of death in the form of these terminal patients. "[T]hese physicians are engaged in a quite common maneuver of turning away from victims, of refusing to listen to their pain, of imposing a regime of silence on them so powerful that even their agonized cries cannot be heard. . . . It requires an act of will to acknowledge this injustice; denial is the path of least resistance, the easy and tempting path." Burt, *Death Is That Man.*

Chapter 4
THE INFORMAL CURRICULUM

89 *young doctors cease being laypeople:* There is a host of books and articles that examine the transformative effects of the hidden curriculum. Some are written from an insider's perspective. Conrad,

"Learning to Doctor"; Klass, *Not Entirely Benign Procedure;* Konner, *Becoming a Doctor;* Rothman, *White Coat.* Others are from an academic point of view. Feudtner et al., "Ethical Erosion"; Griffith and Wilson, "Loss of Student Idealism"; Hafferty and Franks, "Hidden Curriculum"; Ludmerer, *Time to Heal;* Ratanawongsa et al., "Third-Year Medical Students' Experiences." Researchers have also documented similar hidden curricula in medical education outside the United States. Lempp and Seale, "Hidden Curriculum."

94   *concentrating instead on the "treatment algorithm":* While palliative care is a comprehensive approach that can minimize all illness-related suffering, most algorithms for diseases, even terminal ones, fail to mention palliation. Mast et al. recently reviewed the official guidelines for treating nine chronic diseases, all of which typically result in death. While over 90 percent of these guidelines mentioned death, dying, end of life, mortality, or terminal illness, only a little over a third contained any mention of palliation or hospice. Mast et al., "End-of-Life Content." The American Hospice Foundation Guidelines Committee recently published a template to assist guideline writers, specialty groups, and institutions in incorporating palliative care. L. Emanuel et al., "Integrating Palliative Care." Whether they do and to what extent remains to be seen.

95   *These lessons are so powerful:* Billings and Block, "Palliative Care."

95   *"So long as appropriate emotional support":* S. Block and Billings, "Nurturing Humanism." Others have also articulated this belief— that as long as there is guidance or mentorship, the emotional experiences of dealing with the dying prepare doctors to be humane and compassionate clinicians. MacLeod, "On Reflection."

96   *By its very nature, the informal curriculum:* Gorman et al. recently published an excellent review of the effects of the informal curriculum on residents' attitudes toward end-of-life care decisions. Gorman et al., "End-of-life Decision Making."

96   *"assess just what messages":* Hafferty, "Beyond Curriculum Reform."

96   *now require exposure to and knowledge of palliative care:* Morrison and Meier recently published an excellent review article on the clinical practice of palliative care. Morrison and Meier, "Palliative Care." The term "palliative care" was coined by Canadian surgeon Balfour Mount. Dunn, "Surgical Palliative Care." The World Health Organization, the United Nations special agency for health, defines palliative care as "an approach that improves the quality of life of patients and their families facing the problem associated with life-

threatening illness, through the prevention and relief of suffering by means of early identification and impeccable assessment and treatment of pain and other problems, physical, psychosocial, and spiritual." World Health Organization, "Definition." Palliative care is also the "academic, medically mainstream discipline that attempts to integrate the hospice approach into oncology and other areas of clinical medicine from the earliest phases of diagnosis and treatment . . . [and] entertains all appropriate forms of care at any phase of an illness." Choi and Billings, "Changing Perspectives."

The professional association the Academy of Hospice Physicians was created in 1988 (later becoming the American Academy of Hospice and Palliative Medicine), and in 1995 the American Board of Hospice and Palliative Medicine was founded. This group has offered certification since 1996, and more than two thousand physicians have passed the certification exam. Foley, "Palliative Care"; Henig, "Good Death."

While palliative medicine has been a recognized specialty in the United Kingdom since 1987, the American Board of Medical Specialities did not recognize the specialty of Hospice and Palliative Care Medicine until September 2006. The delay has been due in part to differing opinions among palliative care experts, some of whom acknowledge the greater visibility and stature but remain concerned that such specialization could prevent full integration into clinical practice, as has been the case with existing specialties.

96   *In the last five years the American College of Surgeons:* Dunn, "Surgical Palliative Care"; Huffman, "Educating Surgeons." Several surgeons are now focusing their efforts on improving surgical palliative care, most notably Dr. Gregory Dunn. Dunn, "Surgery and Palliative Medicine"; Dunn and Milch, "Introduction and Historical Background"; McCahill et al., "Palliative Surgery"; McCahill et al., "Palliative Outcomes"; Molmenti and Dunn, "Transplantation and Palliative Care."

96   *the surgeons' task force began enrolling residents:* A series of articles published in the *Journal of the American College of Surgeons* documents the work of the task force, including the implementation of end-of-life care education into surgical residency programs. Surgeons Palliative Care Workgroup, "Report from the Field"; McCahill et al., "Palliation."

97   *I discovered guidelines published in 2002:* CDC, *Guideline for Hand Hygiene.*

98   *As the SUPPORT study showed:* SUPPORT Principal Investigators, "SUPPORT Study."

Chapter 5
M AND M

106   *In the early 1970s:* Bosk, *Forgive and Remember;* Bosk, "Occupational Rituals."

106   *"for witnessing [these errors]":* Bosk, *Forgive and Remember.*

107   *always the passive voice and delivered as flatly as possible:* Sociologist Renée Anspach asserts that the manner in which physicians present patients reveals much about professional socialization and medical culture. Case presentations are linguistic rituals that "employ a stylized vocabulary and syntax which reveal tacit and subtle assumptions, beliefs, and values concerning patients, medical knowledge, and medical practice to which physicians in training are covertly socialized." Use of the passive voice, for example, places emphasis on the action or observation described, rather than the agent, usually another physician or nurse. In the case of an action or decision, the passive voice mitigates responsibility; with observations, it lends authority. Anspach, "Sociology of Medical Discourse." Apker and Eggly write that Morning Report—a regular conference in internal medicine departments devoted to case discussions among residents, chief residents, and faculty members— also influences nascent professional identity in trainees. There, the discourse "produces and reproduces systems of domination that privilege scientific medicine and marginalize humanistic approaches." Apker and Eggly, "Communicating Professional Identity." Haber and Lingard write that the way in which medical students learn to present—through trial and error and modeling rather than explicit explanation—increases "the potential for inappropriate and unintended value acquisition." Students misinterpret and infer certain value judgments from indirect feedback. Haber and Lingard, "Oral Presentation Skills."

107   *the responsibility for the error:* Gawande et al. recently analyzed errors reported by surgeons and found that the "vast majority of errors did not appear to be solely the result of individual failure." More often, errors involved more than one clinician and a chain of events that occurred over several phases of care. Gawande et al., "Analysis of Errors." However, surgeons will easily acknowledge

that the "unspoken message is that surgeons are expected to assume personal responsibility for their patients' outcomes; those who look to other factors may not have the ethic of personal responsibility expected in the mature surgeon." Roberson et al., "Morbidity and Mortality Conference."

107 *Rather, it is that horrible sense:* In 1985 Gabbard published a paper on the compulsive personalities of physicians. He wrote that doubt, guilt feelings, and an exaggerated sense of responsibility "seem to form a triad of compulsiveness that characterizes the physician's psychological makeup." While some of these personality traits may be desirable—for example, the conscientious physician who goes "the extra mile" to help a patient—they can also be maladaptive for the doctor, as when, for example, "whatever happens to one's patient [becomes] the physician's responsibility." Gabbard, "Compulsiveness in the Normal Physician."

This sense of personal responsibility is particularly strong in younger physicians. Jackson et al. examined physician descriptions of emotionally powerful patient deaths. They found that for doctors in training, "the type of death, the intensity of emotion or the degree of suffering were new, disturbing, and often overinterpreted to be the result of personal failure." Unfortunately, there is little guidance for these young doctors, and most of these deaths are experienced in isolation. Jackson et al., "Powerful Patient Deaths."

119 *Unfortunately, the very rituals:* Robert Hertz wrote the earliest anthropological study of ritual in death. His work, originally published in 1907, analyzed funerary practices in Borneo in the early twentieth century. Hertz, *Death and the Right Hand.*

119 *"Whatever mental adjustments":* Metcalf and Huntington, *Celebrations of Death.*

119 *Death is rendered optional:* DelVecchio Good et al. studied physician narratives about patient deaths, interviewing internists who practiced in two academic medical centers. These internists also viewed patient deaths as related in some way to their clinical decisions. "[T]hey puzzle over choices gone awry and question the latest inherently risky treatments that may be utilized at the end of patients' lives. Through the interviews, physicians revisit clinical decisions and actions that their colleagues performed." DelVecchio Good et al., "Narrative Nuances."

120 *One of the key vehicles for this change:* M and M has been called "arguably one of our most powerful teaching tools." Harbison and

Regehr, "Faculty and Resident Opinions." It has also been referred to as "the golden hour of surgical education." Gordon, *Morbidity and Mortality Conference.* Several surgical educators have suggested that M and M could serve as a vehicle for changing the current paradigm of surgical education. Gordon, "Surgical Education"; Murayama et al., "Morbidity and Mortality Conference"; Risucci et al., "Assessing Educational Validity"; Roberson et al., "Morbidity and Mortality Conference"; Veldenz et al., "Morbidity and Mortality Conference."

120   *Internal medicine training programs:* While M and M has traditionally been considered a surgical conference, the Accreditation Council for Graduate Medical Education has required this conference in internal medicine residency programs since 1983. Liu, "Error in Medicine." Internal medicine educators, like surgeons, are also working to restructure and redefine the role of M and M in education. Orlander et al., "Learning from Error"; Orlander and Fincke, "Morbidity and Mortality Conference"; Pierluissi et al., "Discussion of Medical Errors"; Schwartz et al., "Medical Residents' Perceptions."

Chapter 6

THE VISIBLE WOMAN

132   *To do otherwise would be to admit:* MacLeod wrote of doctors discussing such "turning points": "[H]alf of the respondents wept as they recounted their stories. . . . The doctors seemed to lower their defensive barriers, and open themselves up to a personal vulnerability that remained alive, despite the passage of years." MacLeod, "On Reflection."

132   *In 1992, as part of a lecture:* Aoun, "Eye of the Storm."

132   *"had turned him into an emaciated, wheelchair-bound":* Ibid.

133   *"It hit me violently that I had lost sight":* Ibid.

133   *"The mystery was solved":* Lerner, "Ultimate Sacrifice."

133   *And on the day after his talk was published:* Ibid.

134   *I have read Hacib Aoun's speech:* Several physicians have written about becoming patients. Bowes, "Doctor as Patient"; English, "Piece of my Mind"; Fromme and Billings, "Dying Doctor"; Haefner, "It's a Boy!"; Horn, "The Other Side"; Mullan, "Seasons of Survival"; Poulson, "Bitter Pills"; Selzer, *Raising the Dead;* Spiro and Mandell, "When Doctors Get Sick"; Terkel, "Dr. Sharon Sandell." Others have described the difficult experience of watching their loved ones become ill. Berwick, "Quality Comes Home"; Chen et al.,

"Role Conflicts"; Chen et al., "Personal Experiences." While Aoun became an eloquent advocate of improved occupational health and end-of-life care, some physicians may have difficulty with the loss of control that occurs. Bedell et al., "Stress of Hospitalization." On a certain level, some may even feel betrayed by "the unconscious pact with the Creator that many physicians have made—we will take care of the sick and You will guarantee us good health." Spiro and Mandell, "When Doctors Get Sick."

134   *We need to devote*: Aoun, "Eye of the Storm."

135   *The recommendations from the resulting work:* Flexner, *Medical Education.*

135   *The Flexner Report influenced over a century:* Beck, "Flexner Report."

136   *instead, it was grounded in problem-based learning:* Peters et al., "New Pathway Program."

136   *A little over a decade later:* Ibid.

136   *Since 1985 other medical schools:* Some of these programs have taken an interdisciplinary approach to medical education. By bringing together students from different disciplines—for example, medicine and social work—these courses bring new perspectives to members of each discipline and promote a better understanding of interdisciplinary professional collaboration. Fineberg et al., "Interdisciplinary Education."

136   *This new approach to medical education:* However, as Robins et al. write, "After a medical school has achieved curricular reform, an even greater challenge presents itself: sustaining the reform." Maintaining these innovations requires faculty support, ongoing program reviews, and institutional commitment of resources. Robins et al., "Sustaining Curricular Reforms."

136   *"that good physician who would say":* Aoun, "Eye of the Storm."

137   *"Because it is particularly":* Ibid.

138   *"I'm excited because I think other people can learn from my experience":* I have witnessed the extraordinary generosity of many patients at the end of life. This "generativity"—the contribution to the well-being of others—may be an important factor in dying well. Steinhauser et al. recently published a study where they conducted focus groups and in-depth interviews of physicians, nurses, social workers, chaplains, hospice volunteers, patients, and recently bereaved family members. The participants identified the major components of a good death. Four of these—pain and symptom management, clear decision making, preparation for death, and

completion—were already well described in the palliative care literature; but two were unexpected—affirmation of the whole person and contributing to others. Steinhauser et al., "A Good Death."

138 *I thought of their lives for the last decade:* In a recent large-scale study, over 85 percent of terminally ill patients required some assistance. Over 70 percent of these patients relied either exclusively or in part on family and friends, many of whom were required to provide skilled nursing and personal care. Of note as well, women provided almost three quarters of all care. E. J. Emanuel et al., "Assistance from Family Members."

139 *and in the end they sat there:* Several studies have documented the profound impact—emotional, physical, and financial—of serious illness on patient families. E. J. Emanuel et al., "Economic and Other Burdens"; Grunfeld et al., "Caring for Elderly." While 90 percent of Americans believe that families should provide care for the terminally ill, the burden usually falls on a few individuals, and as many as 40 percent of families become impoverished as a result. Covinsky et al., "Serious Illness"; E.J. Emanuel et al., "Assistance from Family Members"; L.L. Emanuel et al., "Gaps in End-of-Life Care."

Chapter 7
FIRST, DO NO HARM

146 The Doctor, *first exhibited in 1891:* Shafer, "Art Annotations."

146 *"to put on record":* Ibid.

146 *Fildes and his contemporaries had been witness:* Angier, "Century-Old Death Records."

155 *We wanted to do everything for this child:* Pediatric patients with terminal diseases pose several unique issues, and as Hilden et al. note in their recent survey of 228 pediatric oncologists, there is "a strikingly high reliance on trial and error in learning to care for dying children." Hilden et al., "Attitudes and Practices." While the pediatric oncologists surveyed reported a dearth of formal courses on pediatric palliative care and a lack of accessible palliative care teams or pain services, several health care and advocacy organizations, including the World Health Organization and Children's Hospice International, are working to make palliative care a priority for children with terminal diseases.

156 *Patients now sometimes subject themselves to therapy:* Finucane, "Gravely Ill Becomes Dying."

156   *Cancer patients enrolled in Phase I trials:* It is important to note that participation in a Phase I trial does not necessarily mean that little attention will be paid to the patient's comfort and quality of life. It is possible to enroll in a Phase I trial while simultaneously receiving palliative care measures. NCCN, "Clinical Practice Guidelines"; Meyers and Linder, "Simultaneous Care." End-of-life care specialists believe that such trials would be unethical otherwise. Kapo and Casarett, "Phase I Trials."

156   *Nonetheless, in two recent studies:* C. Daugherty et al., "Perceptions of Cancer Patients"; Meropol et al., "Phase I Cancer Clinical Trials."

157   *And pulling back therapy:* Von Gunten et al. published a paper delineating seven steps to help physicians in end-of-life conversations and asserting that communication skills are particularly important when there are conflicts about futility. They write: "Two powerful motivators for human behavior are guilt and unfinished personal business." Von Gunten et al., "Patient-Physician Relationship."

157   *Many doctors witness firsthand:* Caring for overly treated patients frequently has long-term emotional consequences on physicians as well. Doctors often describe these patient cases in conflictual terms, have difficulty with emotional closure, and end up with long-term anger and frustration. Jackson et al., "Powerful Patient Deaths."

157   *When asked what they would request:* Carmel, "Life-Sustaining Treatments"; Marik et al., "Physicians' Own Preferences."

157   *These physicians are likely to support:* There are also those patients who choose to continue aggressive treatment in the face of terminal illnesses. As Dr. Paul Rousseau, a member of the editorial board of the *Journal of Palliative Medicine*, writes: "[W]hile dying patients may choose treatments deemed futile by professional caregivers, we are compelled to maintain humility and understanding and remain with them throughout their journey with terminal illness. We must allow their autonomy within our own personal boundaries of ethics and morals, and try and guide them to what we perceive as rational palliative therapies when possible, but remain vigilant of our own frustrations and paternalistic attitudes when they choose aggressive treatment." Rousseau, "Aggressive Treatment."

157   *In a recent study:* Solomon et al., "Life-Sustaining Treatments." Medical students, too, find that clinical decisions at the end of life are among the most ethically challenging. Huijer et al., "Medical Students' Cases."

158   *However, only roughly a fifth of all Americans have prepared:* E. J.

ity and Attitudes"; Phipps et al., "Approaching the End of Life."

158 *White Americans, for example:* Phipps et al., "Approaching the End of Life."

158 *And contrary to popular belief:* Burt and others have suggested that the failure of advance directives may have to do with their emphasis on patient autonomy and the difficult realities of exercising individual choice in these matters. Burt, "End of Autonomy"; Kaufman, *A Time to Die.* Writes Burt: "The crucial impetus for the modern embrace of the autonomy framework for terminally ill patients was mistrust of physicians, based on a belief that they regularly disregarded the wishes and interests of their dying patients by pursuing aggressive, painful therapies with no realistic possibility of success, by withholding effective pain relief generally, and by abandoning their patients when death became patently unavoidable. The equivalent dangers in the autonomy framework arise from the practical reluctance of most people to exercise choice." Burt, "End of Autonomy."

158   *there are few differences between patients:* Several studies have shown
       that advance directives can have little impact on care at the end
       of life. Alemayehu et al., "Variability in Physicians' Decisions";
       Goodlin et al., "Death in the Hospital"; Hwang et al., "Outpatient
       End-of-Life Care"; Lee et al., "Clinical Palliative Care." In a recent
       study, even patients with the designation "comfort measures only"
       had as many symptoms at the end of life as other patients. Goodlin
       et al., "Death in the Hospital." It is, as Lee et al. write, a "toss-up."
       Lee et al., "Clinical Palliative Care."

159   *There can also be significant differences:* Even when a patient desig-
       nates a proxy, there can be, for various reasons, discrepancies
       between what the proxy decides and what the patient might have
       wanted. E. J. Emanuel and L. L. Emanuel, "Good Death"; L. L.
       Emanuel and E. J. Emanuel, "Decisions at the End of Life." Physi-
       cians who are patients are not necessarily better at communicat-
       ing their own end-of-life wishes; in a recent study, nearly three
       quarters of physicians reported that their spouses or others were
       aware of their desires, but fewer than a third actually discussed their
       preferences with their own doctors. Gallo et al., "Life-Sustaining
       Treatments."

159   *In one study, 46 percent:* Phipps et al., "Approaching the End of
       Life."

159   *Physicians, too, may be poor judges:* Advance directives may not be
       in the hospital records; physicians may not be aware of and may not
       have discussed the directives with patients; or hospital staff may
       simply ignore patient preferences. E. J. Emanuel and L. L. Emanuel,
       "Good Death"; Frank et al., "Determining Resuscitation Prefer-
       ences." Moreover, advance care planning is often inadequate even
       when physicians believe they are comfortable or knowledgeable
       about the topic. Alpert and Emanuel, "Comparing Utilization";
       Buss et al., "Assessing Competence"; Tulsky et al., "Medical Resi-
       dents Discuss Resuscitation"; Tulsky et al., "Discussing Do-Not-
       Resuscitate Orders"; Tulsky et al., "Opening the Black Box."
       Instead of being a "process of structured discussion and documenta-
       tion woven into the regular process of health care that is reviewed
       and updated on a regular basis," most of these discussions take
       place once and are never revisited again. L. L. Emanuel et al.,
       "Advance Care Planning."

159   *For example, physicians have widely varying interpretations of the
       DNR:* As La Puma et al. write, " '[D]o not resuscitate' means differ-
       ent things to different physicians." La Puma et al., "Life-Sustaining

Treatment." Individual physician attitudes and beliefs regarding DNR affect the way in which they present these options to families and in turn influence the patient's and family's decision. Ventres et al., "Do-Not-Resuscitate Discussions."

159 *doctors and nurses may interpret DNR:* One way in which members of a medical team may interpret DNR orders is through "limited codes" or "slow codes." During these limited codes, physicians might use drugs without chest compressions or abort the code sooner than usual. These can be largely symbolic gestures and tend to occur when there is conflict between physicians or with family members regarding the patient's situation and goals. The physicians who elect to run a limited code do so believing that a patient is near death or will not benefit from further treatment or cardiopulmonary resuscitation because of irreversible brain damage or significant deterioration in quality of life. Muller, "Shades of Blue."

159 *Even with the best medical predictors:* Finucane, "Gravely Ill Becomes Dying." Clinicians also tend to overestimate survival. Glare et al., "Physicians' Survival Predictions." One study compared the average of two trainees' (a resident and a more senior fellow) prognostic judgments with that of an experienced attending physician. The averaged judgment of the two trainees turned out to be slightly more reliable. Poses et al., "House Officers' Prognostic Judgments."

160 *It is a process:* L. L. Emanuel has proposed using a more accurately descriptive asymptotic model of death. Rather than defining two discrete states, life and death, the asymptotic model "builds on the fundamental assertion that both biological life and personhood decline in a continuous fashion rather than as an event." L. L. Emanuel, "Reexamining Death."

160 *"Perhaps the classification":* Lynn and Harrold, *Handbook for Mortals.* Joanne Lynn has written that while health care and life expectancy have changed, the language we use to describe illness, treatment, and even payment has become misleading. Reform in end-of-life care requires that we rethink our perceptions and assumptions. Lynn, "Living Long in Fragile Health." "Often our mental models, categories, and language need updating in order to enable needed reforms." Lynn, *Sick to Death.*

160 *The process of dying can be cast:* Hospice has an important, albeit unfulfilled, role in easing the dying process; some experts in end-of-life care have likened dying without hospice to having surgery

without anesthesia. C.K. Daugherty and Steensma, "Overcoming Obstacles." In 1974, drawing upon the work of Dame Cicely Saunders in England and Elisabeth Kübler-Ross, Dr. Sylvia Lack and Florence Wald, former dean at the Yale University School of Nursing, worked together to establish the first American hospice in Branford, Connecticut. Webb, *The Good Death.* By 1982 hospice was a Medicare benefit. There are now more than 3,600 hospice programs in the United States, but physicians and patients continue to enroll late in the course of disease. While the median length of stay is twenty-two days, more than a third of patients died in seven days or less. While patients and their families may believe that they enrolled in hospice at the right time, palliative care experts remain concerned that they are unable to benefit fully from the programs available. Christakis and Feudtner, "Survival of Medicare Patients"; Kapo et al., "Referring Patients to Hospice"; NHPCO, "2004 Facts and Figures."

Chapter 8
SORRY TO INFORM YOU

165   *I had my only lesson on talking with patients:* Other doctors have similar recollections regarding their training. Terkel, "Dr. John Barrett." Jerome Groopman, who trained nearly two decades before me, writes of his own experience: "[D]uring my nine years of medical school and professional training in the 1970s, I was never instructed in how to speak about dying to a gravely ill patient and the patient's family." Groopman, "Dying Words." In a 1998 study of nearly seven hundred oncologists, fewer than 5 percent had received any formal training in giving patients bad news. Baile et al., "Discussing Disease Progression."

165   *Conversing with patients seemed like an obviously natural skill:* My initial response to the topic of physician-patient conversations was not out of the ordinary. In a 1991 study of 69 internists and their 485 clinic patients, physicians and patients disagreed on the relative importance of effective communication. While they all agreed that the most important aspect of outpatient care is clinical skill and the least important the office environment, patients ranked effective communication second while physicians ranked it sixth. Laine et al., "Elements of Outpatient Care." I was also not alone in regard to how easy I thought these skills would be to acquire—that anyone could

do it well after watching a couple of times. In learning to discuss advance directives with patients, for example, trainees "may cognitively grasp an appropriate approach to communication without possessing the skills to carry it out" and then erroneously believe they need no further training. Tulsky et al., "Discussing Do-Not-Resuscitate Orders."

170 *Bad news thus occurs not just once:* Baile et al., "Discussing Disease Progression"; DelVecchio Good et al., "Discourse on Hope."

170 *I would know how to word terrible news:* While almost all physicians now approach patient conversation with the intent of full disclosure, that practice was not so commonplace a few generations ago. In 1961, 90 percent of physicians preferred not to tell their patients about a cancer diagnosis; by 1979, 98 percent of physicians would choose to do so. Novack et al., "Changes in Physicians' Attitudes"; Oken, "Medical Attitudes."

170 *But these conversations never got easy:* Dickinson and Tournier published a longitudinal study of physician attitudes toward death and terminally ill patients. They found that after a decade of practice, physicians found informing a patient about a terminal diagnosis became less difficult, but there was more discomfort in dealing with dying patients and more anxiety over death. Dickinson and Tournier, "Decade Beyond." In a later paper, the authors found that even after twenty years of practice, physicians still experienced discomfort when dealing with dying patients. Dickinson et al., "Twenty Years Beyond."

170 *One would assume, then:* Over the course of a career, an oncologist will, according to one estimate, deliver bad news to patients approximately twenty thousand times. Zuger, "Doctors Learn."

170 *A recent study:* Gattellari et al., "Treatment Goal."

170 *In another study, again of oncologists:* Unfortunately, physicians' self-assessment affects their practice. In a recent study, those physicians who had a more positive assessment of their knowledge of end-of-life care were also more likely to refer their terminal patients for hospice care. Bradley et al., "Physicians' Ratings."

170 *To compensate for this failure:* American Society of Clinical Oncology, "Remaining Challenges." Meier et al. posit that this "unexamined redoubling of therapeutic efforts" is one of the many signs of unrecognized emotional stress in clinicians. Meier et al., "Inner Life of Physicians." In another recent study, E. J. Emanuel et al. noted that 23 percent of Medicare beneficiaries who died of cancer in

Massachusetts received chemotherapy in the last three months of life and 9 percent in the last month. While those with tumors considered unresponsive to chemotherapy were as likely as patients with chemotherapy-sensitive tumors to receive treatment, the decreasing percentages of patients treated overall do seem to indicate that oncologists exhibit some selectivity in therapy. E. J. Emanuel et al., "Chemotherapy Use."

170 *The health care system has become highly specialized:* In addition, the medical system has incorporated multiple models of accountability in the last couple of decades, ranging from the "traditional professional model" of accountability—focusing on competence and legal and ethical conduct—to the "economic model," where medicine is considered a commodity. In the current managed care climate, these models are often conflated—physicians are required to be caring professionals while carrying the burden of efficient economic productivity—thus causing further confusion in patient care. E. J. Emanuel and L. L. Emanuel, "Preserving Community."

170 *With half a dozen doctors:* Donaldson and Field, "Measuring Quality of Care." What is particularly poignant is that patients want their doctors to discuss these issues with them. Most patients have thought about end-of-life issues, particularly in regard to surrogate decision makers and life-sustaining treatment, but over 50 percent of them want their physicians to bring up the matter first. Lo et al., "Discussing Life-Sustaining Treatment."

171 *Another complicating factor:* S. D. Block and Billings, "Requests to Hasten Death"; DelVecchio Good et al., "Discourse on Hope"; Dias et al., "Breaking Bad News." Additionally, the location of the conversation may have an impact on the quality of the conversation. In one study, patients who were told about their diagnosis of cancer either in the recovery room or over the phone tended to describe the event in more negative terms than those who were told their diagnosis in a hospital room or in a doctor's office. Lind et al., "Telling the Diagnosis."

In another study, researchers found that the more family members spoke during conferences with physicians, the more satisfied they were with physician communication. McDonagh et al., "Family Satisfaction."

171 *Some patients associate these topics with cultural stigmas:* Blackhall et al., "Ethnicity and Attitudes Towards Life Sustaining Technology"; Blackhall et al., "Attitudes Toward Patient Autonomy"; Lapine

et al., "When Cultures Clash." Even within cultural groups, there can be wide variations in how much patients want to be informed. Yun et al., "Disclosure in Terminal Illness."

Medical anthropologists have studied the interplay between culture and illness, and their work has helped illuminate the ways in which culture influences the experience of illness, the language used to report it, treatment decisions, doctor-patient interactions, the relationship between risk factors and social supports, and even the particular environments that may affect physiological reactions and the gene expression of certain diseases. Kleinman, "Culture and Depression"; Kuriyama, *Expressiveness of the Body.* The Institute of Medicine and the American Medical Association have more recently underscored the need for "cultural competence" among practicing physicians. Betancourt, "Cultural Competence." As difficult as this competence may be to attain, it is further complicated by the fact that culture is not fixed but fluid. Kleinman, "Culture and Depression."

171 *others, in an attempt to appear dignified:* Terminally ill patients deal with difficult medical and psychosocial issues, including depression. It can be extraordinarily challenging for physicians to differentiate between "normal" patient adjustment and clinical depression, and time constraints only exacerbate an already difficult situation. S. D. Block, "Consensus Panel."

172 *For doctors, responding appropriately:* Wenrich et al., "Communicating with Dying Patients." A recent article on discussing difficult news in the outpatient oncology clinic likened the situation to the universal precautions against infectious diseases taken by physicians. "History has taught us, tragically, that it is not possible to predict which patients bear communicable, potentially fatal illnesses and that we must prepare for all interactions with patients and their bodily fluids with the awareness that this is a possibility. In a similar manner, oncologists should be trained to be ready to deal with the communication of bad news in virtually all interactions with cancer patients and their families." Eggly et al., "Discussing Bad News."

172 *and at worst extremely time-consuming:* Delbanco writes about a systematic "Patient's Review" that can be incorporated into the traditional medical history and physical exam. This review—a series of thoughtful questions that elicit patient values, fears, and hopes—encourages patients and doctors "to confront and express individual

preferences and values while offering patients a structured opportunity to participate actively in their care." Unfortunately, the biggest obstacle to incorporating this "Patient's Review" is, once again, time. T. L. Delbanco, "Doctor-Patient Relationship."

172 *And time in the hospital:* Rappaport et al. showed in their study that work constraints limit the amount of time surgical residents can spend with the families of terminally ill patients. Rappaport et al., "Surgical Residency."

174 *I learned how to "turf":* Christakis and Feudtner posit that turfing marginalizes psychosocial issues and is a strategy trainees use to deal with their transient, time-limited relationships with patients, families, and other care providers. D.A. Christakis and Feudtner, "Temporary Matters."

181 *As in previous studies:* Back, "Patient-Physician Communication."

181 *In the grand schedule of things:* Razavi et al., "Physicians' Communication Skills."

181 *"Who has got the time?":* The importance of time in improving physician-patient interactions has been noted over and over again in the professional literature. Huffman, "Educating Surgeons"; Larson and Tobin, "End-of-Life Conversations." Drs. Ezekiel and Linda Emanuel write about four models of the physician-patient relationship and advocate the thoughtful and compassionate "deliberative model" while noting that "developing a deliberative physician-patient relationship requires a considerable amount of time." E. J. Emanuel and L. L. Emanuel, "Four Models." Dr. Thomas Delbanco has also published an eloquent piece on how our lack of time in medicine may improve if we listen and do "some serious work hand in hand with those we serve." T. Delbanco, "Breaking Down the Walls."

181 *In that context, five minutes:* Tulsky et al. published a study of physician-patient conversations regarding advance directives. They found that the average conversation was 5.6 minutes. While the content of these conversations might have been less than adequate, the time afforded was actually a large proportion of the average fifteen-to-twenty-minute office visit. Tulsky et al., "Opening the Black Box."

182 *Over the last five years, training programs:* Several studies have documented the effect of extended work hours in residency training. The resultant fatigue in young doctors increases not only attentional failures and medical errors but also the risk of motor vehicle accidents outside the hospital. Barger et al., "Extended Work Shifts";

Landrigan et al., "Reducing Interns' Work Hours"; Lockley et al., "Reducing Interns' Weekly Work."

182 *the change has had some unpredictable repercussions:* Since July 2003, the Accreditation Council for Graduate Medical Education has had resident work-hour regulations in place for all specialties. To adjust to these decreased resident work hours, patient care is now parceled out in shifts, with teams of residents transferring the care of patients at the end of each shift. The ultimate outcome of these changes remains unclear. While there are reports of improvements in certain aspects of patient care, such as resident-nursing communication and faster identification of patient problems, it has been difficult to evaluate patient perceptions and the impact of shift-type work on continuity of care and medical education. Gawande et al., "Analysis of Errors"; Goldstein et al., "Night-Float System"; Lowenstein, "Limitations on Resident Work"; Mukherjee, "Precarious Exchange."

182 *The transient physician-patient relationships of residency:* Christakis and Feudtner also argue that these transient relationships during residency training are detrimental to the emotional and ethical development of young doctors. D.A. Christakis and Feudtner, "Temporary Matters."

182 *This constant tension:* Medical students in the earliest phases of their clinical education began to feel a sense of time urgency. Rappaport and Witzke, in their study of medical students during third-year rotations, noted that the overwhelming majority of medical students believed that certain specialties had differing time constraints, and those constraints resulted in less time to spend with the terminally ill. Rappaport and Witzke, "Clinical Years of Medical School."

182 *"Doctors' anguish":* Zuger, "Dissatisfaction with Medical Practice."

182 *A terrible sequence unfolds:* In a 1991 survey of almost six hundred practicing medical oncologists, nearly 60 percent reported experiencing burnout, and the most frequent reason was frustration or a sense of failure. Whippen and Canellos, "Burnout Syndrome." Meier et al. believe that in caring for the seriously ill, physicians exhibit a wide range of emotional responses, many of which go ignored. This lack of self-examination contributes to high rates of burnout, depression, and substance abuse in clinicians. Meier et al., "Inner Life of Physicians." Others have also studied the increased vulnerability of physicians to problems such as depression, substance abuse, marital problems, and even suicide. Miller and McGowen, "Painful Truth."

182   *A group of researchers recently looked at burnout:* McManus et al., "Stress, Burnout and Doctors' Attitudes."

183   *"just as genes are not destiny":* Ibid.

Chapter 9
THROUGH THE LOOKING GLASS

193   *"The syllogism he had learned":* Tolstoy, *Death of Ivan Ilyich.* Weinstein writes about this novella: "Tolstoy makes us squirm, not only because he exposes the evasiveness of all human pursuits but also because he has the bad taste to lock us into Ilyich's position. . . . [Ilyich] is constantly thinking about the unthinkable, constantly making us think about it, leading us to the horrid conclusion that he is dreadfully logical, that of course we would all obsess about dying if we actually knew it was happening. . . . There is a stench in this brief novella, like a fart in a crowded room, and it reeks of mortality, of somatic thralldom, of a *huis clos* that no one exits." Weinstein, *A Scream Goes Through.*

195   *On average, a physician in training:* Billings and Block, "Palliative Care."

195   *that number would by force seem to make death frighteningly routine:* The young doctor's experience of witnessing so many deaths has been compared to being in a war or natural catastrophe, and the reactions of residents have been likened to post-traumatic stress disorder. Ferris et al., "When the Patient Dies."

202   *I began to write the truth:* Narrative medicine, or literature and medicine, is an emerging field that uses writing, reading, narratives, and the approaches from literary critique as ways in which to improve ourselves as physicians. Charon, "Literature and Medicine"; Charon, "Narrative Medicine"; Charon, "Narrative and Medicine;" Charon et al., "Literature and Medicine"; Spiro and Mandell, "When Doctors Get Sick"; Verghese, "Physician as Storyteller"; Verghese, "Calling." Medical educators are also using narratives in end-of-life care courses. Students express their concerns through writing, and educators then use these pieces to identify topics for discussion that are particularly meaningful to the students. Williams et al., "Medical Education."

206   *researchers continue to find funding support:* The Robert Wood Johnson Foundation created the national Promoting Excellence in End-of-Life Care program in 1997. From 1998 to 2004, the program gave approximately $9.2 million to twenty-two projects aimed at develop-

ing innovative models for delivering palliative care. Byock et al. recently published a report examining the outcome of these projects. In a few years' time, the projects—in populations as diverse as native Alaskans, military veterans, African Americans, inner-city medically underserved, and pediatric patients—appeared to have made significant inroads in end-of-life care. Despite the practical, academic difficulty of measuring quality outcomes at the end of life (Morrison et al., "Improving the Quality of Care"), these twenty-two projects successfully expanded access to and improved the quality of palliative care, yet were economically feasible and acceptable to providers and patients alike. Byock et al., "Promoting Excellence."

206 *Educational opportunities have increased as well:* Hill characterizes education prior to 1995 as a "well-established pattern of neglect of medical education in the care of the dying." Hill, "Treating the Dying."

206 *The number of medical schools:* Over the past decade, some medical school educators have taken innovative approaches to teaching end-of-life care. S. D. Block and Billings, "Learning from the Dying"; Porter-Williamson et al., "Improving Knowledge." And while these courses represent a significant leap forward compared to a generation prior, almost a third of medical students still would like more instruction about death and dying. Barzansky et al., "Education in End-of-Life Care"; Dickinson and Mermann, "Death Education"; Association of American Medical Colleges, *Medical School Graduation Questionnaire.*

206 *the Liaison Committee on Medical Education:* LCME, "Standards for Accreditation." In a recent survey of medical education deans, a majority also supported incorporating more end-of-life care into medical school curricula. Sullivan et al., "Medical Education Deans." Of note as well, in 2001 California became the first state to require that doctors take courses in pain management and palliative care in order to maintain their state medical licensure. Charatan, "New Law."

206 *There have also been significant changes in residency training:* An increasing number of residency training programs have added clinical rotations or courses that focus on end-of-life care. Liao et al., "Innovative, Longitudinal Program"; Stevens et al., "Education, Ethics, and End-of-Life Decisions." Nevertheless, the offerings still fall short of national consensus conference recommendations on end-of-life care education. Weissman and Block, "ACGME Requirements."

206   *The American Board of Internal Medicine:* Weissman and Block, "ACGME Requirements."

206   *Moreover, there are now twenty subspecialty fellowships:* Foley, "Palliative Care."

206   *In June 2006, the American Council of Graduate Medical Education:* American Board of Hospice and Palliative Medicine, "Transition to ABMS Subspecialty."

207   *In a recent survey of one hundred academic medical centers:* Billings and Pantilat, "Survey of Palliative Care." The acute care hospital is a particularly important educational site. Residents and students spend a significant portion of their training in this setting, and as many as 50 percent of patients die there. Weissman et al., "Incorporating Palliative Care Education."

207   *This growth parallels the increase:* Morrison et al., "Growth of Palliative Care."

207   *What is more significant for our patients:* Suffering encompasses not only physical discomfort but also a loss of meaning and purpose in life; physicians need to be able to address that loss however it may manifest in the individual patient. Byock, *Dying Well.* Some would argue that this form of suffering is more significant than physical pain. Frankl in his book *Man's Search for Meaning* recalls his time spent in a Nazi concentration camp; he asserts that loss of meaning and purpose are the true root of human suffering. Frankl, *Search for Meaning.* The physician's ability to be an empathic witness can affirm that sense of meaning for the dying patient, and such empathy is, as Kleinman asserts, "a moral act, not a technical procedure." Kleinman, *Illness Narratives.*

211   *"it was just as he had wished":* Experts in end-of-life care, while advocating dying with dignity, also acknowledge that the definition for each patient and his or her family may be unique. Chochinov, "Dignity-Conserving Care."

BIBLIOGRAPHY

Alemayehu, E., Molloy, D. W., Guyatt, G. H., et al. "Variability in Physicians' Decisions on Caring for Chronically Ill Elderly Patients: An International Study." *Canadian Medical Association Journal* 1991;144(9):1133–38.

Alpert, H. R., Emanuel, L. "Comparing Utilization of Life-Sustaining Treatments with Patient and Public Preferences." *Journal of General Internal Medicine* 1998;13(3):175–81.

American Board of Hospice and Palliative Medicine. "The Transition to an ABMS Subspeciality." 2006 [cited October 4, 2006]; available from: http://www.abhpm.org/gfxc_100.aspx.

American Society of Clinical Oncology. "Largest Survey of Cancer Specialists Finds Physician Education, Access to Services, Patient Depression, Remaining Challenges to Providing Quality End-of-Life Care." Annual Meeting News Release 1998 [cited March 13, 2006]; available from: http://www.asco.org/portal/site/ASCO/menuitem.c543a013502b2a89de 912310320041a0/?vgnextoid=5b618c393c458010VgnVCM100000ed7 30ad1RCRD.

Angier, N. "Century-Old Death Records Provide a Glimpse into Medicine's History." *New York Times*, May 25, 2004.

Anspach, R. R. "Notes on the Sociology of Medical Discourse: The Language of Case Presentation." *Journal of Health and Social Behavior* 1988;29(4):357–75.

Aoun, H. "From the Eye of the Storm, with the Eyes of a Physician." *Annals of Internal Medicine* 1992;116(4):335–38.

Apker, J., Eggly, S. "Communicating Professional Identity in Medical Socialization: Considering the Ideological Discourse of Morning Report." *Qualitative Health Research* 2004;14(3):411–29.

Aries, P. *The Hour of Our Death.* New York: Alfred A. Knopf, 1981.

Association of American Medical Colleges. *2002 Medical School Graduation Questionnaire: All School Report.* Washington, D.C.: Association of American Medical Colleges, 2002.

Back, A. "Patient-Physician Communication in Oncology: What Does the Evidence Show?" *Oncology* 2006;20(1):67–74.

Baile, W. F., Glober, G. A., Lenzi, R., et al. "Discussing Disease Progression and End-of-Life Decisions." *Oncology (Williston Park)* 1999;13(7):1021–31; discussion 1031–38, 1038.

Barger, L. K., Cade, B. E., Ayas, N. T., et al. "Extended Work Shifts and the Risk of Motor Vehicle Crashes Among Interns." *New England Journal of Medicine* 2005;352(2):125–34.

Barzansky, B., Veloski, J. J., Miller, R., et al. "Education in End-of-Life Care During Medical School and Residency Training." *Academic Medicine* 1999;74(10 Suppl):S102–4.

Beck, A. H. "The Flexner Report and the Standardization of American Medical Education." *Journal of the American Medical Association* 2004;291(17):2139–40.

Bedell, S. E., Cleary, P. D., Delbanco, T. L. "The Kindly Stress of Hospitalization." *American Journal of Medicine* 1984;77(4):592–96.

Bertman, S. L., Marks, S. C., Jr. "Humanities in Medical Education: Rationale and Resources for the Dissection Laboratory." *Medical Education* 1985;19(5):374–81.

Berwick, D. M. "Quality Comes Home." *Annals of Internal Medicine* 1996;125(10):839–43.

Betancourt, J. R. "Cultural Competence—Marginal or Mainstream Movement?" *New England Journal of Medicine* 2004;351(10):953–55.

Billings, J. A., Block, S. "Palliative Care in Undergraduate Medical Education. Status Report and Future Directions." *Journal of the American Medical Association* 1997;278(9):733–38.

Billings, J. A., Pantilat, S. "Survey of Palliative Care Programs in United States Teaching Hospitals." *Journal of Palliative Medicine* 2001; 4(3):309–14.

Blackhall, L. J., Frank, G., Murphy, S. T., et al. "Ethnicity and Attitudes Towards Life Sustaining Technology." *Social Science and Medicine* 1999;48(12):1779–89.

Blackhall, L. J., Murphy, S. T., Frank, G., et al. "Ethnicity and Attitudes

Toward Patient Autonomy." *Journal of the American Medical Association* 1995;274(10):820–25.

Block, S. D. "Assessing and Managing Depression in the Terminally Ill Patient. ACP-ASIM End-of-Life Care Consensus Panel. American College of Physicians—American Society of Internal Medicine." *Annals of Internal Medicine* 2000;132(3):209–18.

Block, S. D. "Perspectives on Care at the Close of Life. Psychological Considerations, Growth, and Transcendence at the End of Life: The Art of the Possible." *Journal of the American Medical Association* 2001;285(22):2898–2905.

Block, S. D., Billings, J. A. "Learning from the Dying." *New England Journal of Medicine* 2005;353(13):1313–15.

Block, S. D., Billings, J. A. "Nurturing Humanism Through Teaching Palliative Care." *Academic Medicine* 1998;73(7):763–65.

Block, S. D., Billings, J. A. "Patient Requests to Hasten Death. Evaluation and Management in Terminal Care." *Archives of Internal Medicine* 1994;154(18):2039–47.

Bosk, C. L. *Forgive and Remember: Managing Medical Failure.* Chicago: University of Chicago Press, 1979.

Bosk, C. L. "Occupational Rituals in Patient Management." *New England Journal of Medicine* 1980;303(2):71–76.

Bowes, D. "The Doctor as Patient: An Encounter with Guillain-Barre Syndrome." *Canadian Medical Association Journal* 1984;131(11):1343–48.

Bradley, E. H., Cramer, L. D., Bogardus, S.T., Jr., et al. "Physicians' Ratings of Their Knowledge, Attitudes, and End-of-Life-Care Practices." *Academic Medicine* 2002;77(4):305–11.

Burt, R. A. *Death Is That Man Taking Names: Intersections of American Medicine, Law, and Culture.* Berkeley: University of California Press, 2002.

Burt, R. A. "The End of Autonomy." *Hastings Center Report* 2005;Spec No:S9–13.

Buss, M. K., Alexander, G. C., Switzer, G. E., et al. "Assessing Competence of Residents to Discuss End-of-Life Issues." *Journal of Palliative Medicine* 2005;8(2):363–71.

Byock, I. *Dying Well: The Prospect for Growth at the End of Life.* New York: Riverhead Books, 1997.

Byock, I., Twohig, J. S., Merriman, M., et al. "Promoting Excellence in End-of-Life Care: A Report on Innovative Models of Palliative Care." *Journal of Palliative Medicine* 2006;9(1):137–51.

Carmel, S. "Life-Sustaining Treatments: What Doctors Do, What They

Want for Themselves and What Elderly Persons Want." *Social Science and Medicine* 1999;49(10):1401–8.

Centers for Disease Control and Prevention. *Guideline for Hand Hygiene in Health-Care Settings; Recommendations of the Healthcare Infection Control Practices Advisory Committee and the HICPAC/SHEA/APIC/IDSA Hand Hygiene Task Force.* Atlanta: CDC, October 25, 2002.

Charatan, F. "New Law Requires Doctors to Learn Care of the Dying." *British Medical Journal* 2001;323:1088.

Charon, R. "Literature and Medicine: Origins and Destinies." *Academic Medicine* 2000;75(1):23–27.

Charon, R. "Narrative and Medicine." *New England Journal of Medicine* 2004;350(9):862–64.

Charon, R. "Narrative Medicine: Form, Function, and Ethics." *Annals of Internal Medicine* 2001;134(1):83–87.

Charon, R., Banks, J. T., Connelly, J. E., et al. "Literature and Medicine Contributions." *Annals of Internal Medicine* 1995;122(8):599–606.

Chen, F. M., Feudtner, C., Rhodes, L. A., et al. "Role Conflicts of Physicians and Their Family Members: Rules but no Rulebook." *Western Journal of Medicine* 2001;175(4):236–39; discussion 240.

Chen, F. M., Rhodes, L. A., Green, L. A. "Family Physicians' Personal Experiences of Their Fathers' Health Care." *Journal of Family Practice* 2001;50(9):762–66.

Childress, S. "Invasion of the Body Snatchers." *Newsweek,* March 6, 2006:46.

Chochinov, H. M. "Dignity-Conserving Care—A New Model for Palliative Care: Helping the Patient Feel Valued." *Journal of the American Medical Association* 2002;287(17):2253–60.

Chochinov, H. M., Tataryn, D. J., Wilson, K. G., et al. "Prognostic Awareness and the Terminally Ill." *Psychosomatics* 2000;41(6):500–504.

Choi, Y. S., Billings, J. A. "Changing Perspectives on Palliative Care." *Oncology (Williston Park)* 2002;16(4):515–22.

Christakis, D. A., Feudtner, C. "Temporary Matters. The Ethical Consequences of Transient Social Relationships in Medical Training." *Journal of the American Medical Association* 1997;278(9):739–43.

Christakis, N. A., Escarce, J. J. "Survival of Medicare Patients After Enrollment in Hospice Programs." *New England Journal of Medicine* 1996;335(3):172–78.

Chuck, J. M. "Do Premedical Students Know What They Are Getting Into?" *Western Journal of Medicine* 1996;164(3):228–30.

Conrad, P. "Learning to Doctor: Reflections on Recent Accounts of the

Medical School Years." *Journal of Health and Social Behavior* 1988;29(4):323–32.

Covinsky, K. E., Goldman, L., Cook, E. F., et al. "The Impact of Serious Illness on Patients' Families. SUPPORT Investigators. Study to Understand Prognoses and Preferences for Outcomes and Risks of Treatment." *Journal of the American Medical Association* 1994;272(23):1839–44.

Daugherty, C., Ratain, M. J., Grochowski, E., et al. "Perceptions of Cancer Patients and Their Physicians Involved in Phase I Trials." *Journal of Clinical Oncology* 1995;13(5):1062–72.

Daugherty, C. K., Steensma, D. P. "Overcoming Obstacles to Hospice Care: An Ethical Examination of Inertia and Inaction." *Journal of Clinical Oncology* 2002;20(11):2752–55.

Delbanco, T. "Listening and Breaking Down the Walls." *Literature and Medicine* 2002;21(2):191–200.

Delbanco, T. L. "Enriching the Doctor-Patient Relationship by Inviting the Patient's Perspective." *Annals of Internal Medicine* 1992;116(5): 414–18.

DelVecchio Good, M. J., Gadmer, N. M., Ruopp, P., et al. "Narrative Nuances on Good and Bad Deaths: Internists' Tales from High-Technology Work Places." *Social Science and Medicine* 2004; 58(5):939–53.

DelVecchio Good, M. J., Good, B. J., Schaffer, C., et al. "American Oncology and the Discourse on Hope." *Culture, Medicine, and Psychiatry* 1990;14(1):59–79.

Dias, L., Chabner, B. A., Lynch, T. J., Jr., et al. "Breaking Bad News: A Patient's Perspective." *Oncologist* 2003;8(6):587–96.

Dickinson, G. E., Mermann, A. C. "Death Education in U.S. Medical Schools, 1975–1995." *Academic Medicine* 1996;71(12):1348–49.

Dickinson, G. E., Tournier, R. E. "A Decade Beyond Medical School: A Longitudinal Study of Physicians' Attitudes Toward Death and Terminally-Ill Patients." *Social Science and Medicine* 1994;38(10): 1397–1400.

Dickinson, G. E., Tournier, R. E., Still, B. J. "Twenty Years Beyond Medical School: Physicians' Attitudes Toward Death and Terminally Ill Patients." *Archives of Internal Medicine* 1999;159(15):1741–44.

Diem, S. J., Lantos, J. D., Tulsky, J. A. "Cardiopulmonary Resuscitation on Television. Miracles and Misinformation." *New England Journal of Medicine* 1996;334(24):1578–82.

Donaldson, M. S., Field, M. J. "Measuring Quality of Care at the End of Life." *Archives of Internal Medicine* 1998;158(2):121–28.

Dunn, G. P. "Surgery and Palliative Medicine: New Horizons." *Journal of Palliative Medicine* 1998;1(3):215–19.

Dunn, G. P. "Surgical Palliative Care: An Enduring Framework for Surgical Care." *Surgical Clinics of North America* 2005;85(2):169–90.

Dunn, G. P., Milch, R. A. "Introduction and Historical Background of Palliative Care: Where Does the Surgeon Fit In?" *Journal of the American College of Surgeons* 2001;193(3):325–28.

Dyer, K. A. "Reshaping Our Views of Death and Dying." *Journal of the American Medical Association* 1992;267(9):1265, 1269–70.

Eggly, S., Penner, L., Albrecht, T. L., et al. "Discussing Bad News in the Outpatient Oncology Clinic: Rethinking Current Communication Guidelines." *Journal of Clinical Oncology* 2006;24(4):716–19.

Ellard, J. "The Disease of Being a Doctor." *Medical Journal of Australia* 1974;2(9):318–23.

Emanuel, E. J., Emanuel, L. L. "Four Models of the Physician-Patient Relationship." *Journal of the American Medical Association* 1992;267(16):2221–26.

Emanuel, E. J., Emanuel, L. L. "Preserving Community in Health Care." *Journal of Health Politics, Policy and Law* 1997;22(1):147–84.

Emanuel, E. J., Emanuel, L. L. "The Promise of a Good Death." *Lancet* 1998;351 Suppl 2:SII21–29.

Emanuel, E. J., Fairclough, D. L., Slutsman, J., et al. "Assistance from Family Members, Friends, Paid Care Givers, and Volunteers in the Care of Terminally Ill Patients." *New England Journal of Medicine* 1999;341(13):956–63.

Emanuel, E. J., Fairclough, D. L., Slutsman, J., et al. "Understanding Economic and Other Burdens of Terminal Illness: The Experience of Patients and Their Caregivers." *Annals of Internal Medicine* 2000;132(6):451–59.

Emanuel, E. J., Young-Xu, Y., Levinsky, N. G., et al. "Chemotherapy Use Among Medicare Beneficiaries at the End of Life." *Annals of Internal Medicine* 2003;138(8):639–43.

Emanuel, L., Alexander, C., Arnold, R. M., et al. "Integrating Palliative Care into Disease Management Guidelines." *Journal of Palliative Medicine* 2004;7(6):774–83.

Emanuel, L. L. "Reexamining Death. The Asymptotic Model and a Bounded Zone Definition." *Hastings Center Report* 1995;25(4):27–35.

Emanuel, L. L., Emanuel, E. J. "Decisions at the End of Life. Guided by Communities of Patients." *Hastings Center Report* 1993;23(5):6–14.

Emanuel, L. L., von Gunten, C. F., Ferris, F. D. "Advance Care Planning." *Archives of Family Medicine* 2000;9(10):1181–87.

Emanuel, L. L., von Gunten, C. F., Ferris, F. D. "Gaps in End-of-Life Care." *Archives of Family Medicine* 2000;9(10):1176–80.

English, T. L. "A Piece of My Mind. Skeptical of Skeptics." *Journal of the American Medical Association* 1991;265(8):964.

Ferris, T. G., Hallward, J. A., Ronan, L., et al. "When the Patient Dies: A Survey of Medical Housestaff About Care After Death." *Journal of Palliative Medicine* 1998;1(3):231–39.

Feudtner, C., Christakis, D. A., Christakis, N. A. "Do Clinical Clerks Suffer Ethical Erosion? Students' Perceptions of Their Ethical Environment and Personal Development." *Academic Medicine* 1994;69(8):670–79.

Fineberg, I. C., Wenger, N. S., Forrow, L. "Interdisciplinary Education: Evaluation of a Palliative Care Training Intervention for Pre-Professionals." *Academic Medicine* 2004;79(8):769–76.

Finucane, T. E. "How Gravely Ill Becomes Dying: A Key to End-of-Life Care." *Journal of the American Medical Association* 1999;282(17): 1670–72.

Flexner, A. *Medical Education in the United States and Canada: A Report to the Carnegie Foundation for the Advancement of Teaching.* New York: Carnegie Foundation, 1910.

Foley, K. M. "The Past and Future of Palliative Care." *Hastings Center Report* 2005;Spec No:S42–46.

Fox, R. C. *The Sociology of Medicine: A Participant Observer's View.* Englewood Cliffs, NJ: Prentice Hall, 1989.

Frank, C., Heyland, D. K., Chen, B., et al. "Determining Resuscitation Preferences of Elderly Inpatients: A Review of the Literature." *Canadian Medical Association Journal* 2003;169(8):795–99.

Frankl, V. E. *Man's Search for Meaning.* Boston: Beacon Press, 1992.

Freud, S. *Civilisation, War and Death.* 2nd ed. London: Hogarth Press, 1953.

Fromme, E., Billings, J. A. "Care of the Dying Doctor: On the Other End of the Stethoscope." *Journal of the American Medical Association* 2003;290(15):2048–55.

Gabbard, G. O. "The Role of Compulsiveness in the Normal Physician." *Journal of the American Medical Association* 1985;254(20):2926–29.

Gallo, J. J., Straton, J. B., Klag, M. J., et al. "Life-Sustaining Treatments: What Do Physicians Want and Do They Express Their Wishes to Others?" *Journal of the American Geriatrics Society* 2003;51(7):961–69.

Gattellari, M., Voigt, K. J., Butow, P. N., et al. "When the Treatment Goal Is Not Cure: Are Cancer Patients Equipped to Make Informed Decisions?" *Journal of Clinical Oncology* 2002;20(2):503–13.

Gawande, A. A., Zinner, M. J., Studdert, D. M., et al. "Analysis of Errors

Reported by Surgeons at Three Teaching Hospitals." *Surgery* 2003;133(6):614–21.

Giegerich, S. *Body of Knowledge: One Semester of Gross Anatomy, the Gateway to Becoming a Doctor.* New York: Scribner, 2001.

Glare, P., Virik, K., Jones, M., et al. "A Systematic Review of Physicians' Survival Predictions in Terminally Ill Cancer Patients." *British Medical Journal* 2003;327(7408):195.

Goldstein, M. J., Kim, E., Widmann, W. D., et al. "A 360 Degrees Evaluation of a Night-Float System for General Surgery: A Response to Mandated Work-Hours Reduction." *Current Surgery* 2004;61(5): 445–51.

Goodlin, S. J., Winzelberg, G. S., Teno, J. M., et al. "Death in the Hospital." *Archives of Internal Medicine* 1998;158(14):1570–72.

Gordon, L. A. *Gordon's Guide to the Surgical Morbidity and Mortality Conference.* Philadelphia: Hanley & Belfus, 1994.

Gordon, L. A. "Re: 'Surgical Education: In Need of a Shift in Paradigm.' " *Surgery* 2004;135(2):240.

Gorman, T. E., Ahern, S. P., Wiseman, J., et al. "Residents' End-of-Life Decision Making with Adult Hospitalized Patients: A Review of the Literature." *Academic Medicine* 2005;80(7):622–33.

Griffith, C. H., III, Wilson, J. F. "The Loss of Student Idealism in the 3rd-Year Clinical Clerkships." *Evaluation and the Health Professions* 2001;24(1):61–71.

Groopman, J. "Dying Words: How Should Doctors Deliver Bad News?" *New Yorker,* October 28, 2002:62–70.

Grunfeld, E., Glossop, R., McDowell, I., et al. "Caring for Elderly People at Home: The Consequences to Caregivers." *Canadian Medical Association Journal* 1997;157(8):1101–5.

Haber, R. J., Lingard, L. A. "Learning Oral Presentation Skills: A Rhetorical Analysis with Pedagogical and Professional Implications." *Journal of General Internal Medicine* 2001;16(5):308–14.

Haefner, H. K. "It's a Boy!" *Annals of Internal Medicine* 1994;120(9):806.

Hafferty, F. W. "Beyond Curriculum Reform: Confronting Medicine's Hidden Curriculum." *Academic Medicine* 1998;73(4):403–7.

Hafferty, F. W. "Cadaver Stories and the Emotional Socialization of Medical Students." *Journal of Health and Social Behavior* 1988; 29(4):344–56.

Hafferty, F. W. *Into the Valley: Death and the Socialization of Medical Students.* New Haven: Yale University Press, 1991.

Hafferty, F. W., Franks, R. "The Hidden Curriculum, Ethics Teaching, and

259

the Structure of Medical Education." *Academic Medicine* 1994;69(11):
861–71.

Harbison, S. P., Regehr, G. "Faculty and Resident Opinions Regarding the
Role of Morbidity and Mortality Conference." *American Journal of
Surgery* 1999;177(2):136–39.

Hays, T. "Four Indicted in Alleged Tissue-Theft Scheme." *Hartford
Courant,* February 24, 2006, Sect. A7.

Hendricks, T. "Dying Patients, Kin Want More Aggressive Effort to Relieve
Pain." *San Francisco Chronicle,* May 27, 2001, Sect. A4.

Henig, R. M. "Will We Ever Arrive at the Good Death?" *New York Times
Magazine,* August 7, 2005:26–68.

Hertz, R. *Death and the Right Hand.* With an introduction by E. E. Evans-
Pritchard. Glencoe, IL: Free Press, 1960.

Hilden, J. M., Emanuel, E. J., Fairclough, D. L., et al. "Attitudes and Practices Among Pediatric Oncologists Regarding End-of-Life Care: Results
of the 1998 American Society of Clinical Oncology Survey." *Journal of
Clinical Oncology* 2001;19(1):205–12.

Hill, T. P. "Treating the Dying Patient. The Challenge for Medical Education." *Archives of Internal Medicine* 1995;155(12):1265–69.

Horn, M. O. "The Other Side of the Bed Rail." *Annals of Internal Medicine*
1999;130(11):940–41.

Huffman, J. L. "Educating Surgeons for the New Golden Hours: Honing the
Skills of Palliative Care." *Surgical Clinics of North America*
2005;85(2):383–91.

Huijer, M., van Leeuwen, E., Boenink, A., et al. "Medical Students' Cases
as an Empirical Basis for Teaching Clinical Ethics." *Academic Medicine*
2000;75(8):834–39.

Hwang, J. P., Smith, M. L., Flamm, A. L. "Challenges in Outpatient End-
of-Life Care: Wishes to Avoid Resuscitation." *Journal of Clinical Oncology* 2004;22(22):4643–45.

Jackson, V. A., Sullivan, A. M., Gadmer, N. M., et al. " 'It Was Haunting.'
Physicians' Descriptions of Emotionally Powerful Patient Deaths." *Academic Medicine* 2005;80(7):648–56.

Kagawa-Singer, M., Blackhall, L. J. "Negotiating Cross-Cultural Issues at
the End of Life: 'You Got to Go Where He Lives.' " *Journal of the American Medical Association* 2001;286(23):2993–3001.

Kane, A. C., Hogan, J. D. "Death Anxiety in Physicians: Defensive
Style, Medical Specialty, and Exposure to Death." *Omega*
1985–1986;16(1):11–22.

Kapo, J., Casarett, D. "Palliative Care in Phase I Trials: An Ethical Obligation or Undue Inducement?" *Journal of Palliative Medicine* 2002;5(5):661–65.

Kapo, J., Harrold, J., Carroll, J. T., et al. "Are We Referring Patients to Hospice Too Late? Patients' and Families' Opinions." *Journal of Palliative Medicine* 2005;8(3):521–27.

Kaufman, S. R. *And a Time to Die: How American Hospitals Shape the End of Life.* New York: Scribner, 2005.

Klass, P. *A Not Entirely Benign Procedure.* New York: G. P. Putnam's Sons, 1987.

Kleinman, A. "Culture and Depression." *New England Journal of Medicine* 2004;351(10):951–53.

Kleinman, A. *Patients and Healers in the Context of Culture: An Exploration of the Borderland Between Anthropology, Medicine, and Psychiatry.* Berkeley: University of California Press, 1980.

Kleinman, A. *Social Origins of Distress and Disease: Depression, Neurasthenia, and Pain in Modern China.* New Haven: Yale University Press, 1986.

Kleinman, A. *The Illness Narratives: Suffering, Healing, and the Human Condition.* New York: Basic Books, 1988.

Konner, M. *Becoming a Doctor: A Journey of Initiation in Medical School.* New York: Penguin, 1987.

Kuriyama, S. *The Expressiveness of the Body and the Divergence of Greek and Chinese Medicine.* New York: Zone Books, 1999.

Laine, C., Davidoff, F., Lewis, C. E., et al. "Important Elements of Outpatient Care: A Comparison of Patients' and Physicians' Opinions." *Annals of Internal Medicine* 1996;125(8):640–45.

Landrigan, C. P., Rothschild, J. M., Cronin, J. W., et al. "Effect of Reducing Interns' Work Hours on Serious Medical Errors in Intensive Care Units." *New England Journal of Medicine* 2004;351(18):1838–48.

Lapine, A., Wang-Cheng, R., Goldstein, M., et al. "When Cultures Clash: Physician, Patient, and Family Wishes in Truth Disclosure for Dying Patients." *Journal of Palliative Medicine* 2001;4(4):475–80.

La Puma, J., Silverstein, M. D., Stocking, C. B., et al. "Life-Sustaining Treatment. A Prospective Study of Patients with DNR Orders in a Teaching Hospital." *Archives of Internal Medicine* 1988;148(10):2193–98.

Larson, D. G., Tobin, D. R. "End-of-Life Conversations: Evolving Practice and Theory." *Journal of the American Medical Association* 2000; 284(12):1573–78.

Lee, K. F., Purcell, G. P., Hinshaw, D. B., et al. "Clinical Palliative Care for Surgeons: Part 1." *Journal of the American College of Surgeons* 2004;198(2):303–19.

Lempp, H., Seale, C. "The Hidden Curriculum in Undergraduate Medical Education: Qualitative Study of Medical Students' Perceptions of Teaching." *British Medical Journal* 2004;329(7469):770–73.

Lerner, B. "For a Young Doctor, the Ultimate Sacrifice." *New York Times*, August 24, 2004, Sect. F5.

Liaison Committee on Medical Education. "Functions and Structure of a Medical School: Standards for Accreditation of Medical Education Programs Leading to the M.D. Degree." 2004 (updated 2005) [cited March 16, 2006]; available from: http://www.lcme.org/functions2005oct .pdf.

Liao, S., Amin, A., Rucker, L. "An Innovative, Longitudinal Program to Teach Residents About End-of-Life Care." *Academic Medicine* 2004;79(8):752–57.

Lind, S. E., DelVecchio Good, M. J., Seidel, S., et al. "Telling the Diagnosis of Cancer." *Journal of Clinical Oncology* 1989;7(5):583–89.

Liu, V. "Error in Medicine: The Role of the Morbidity and Mortality Conference." *Virtual Mentor: Ethics Journal of the American Medical Association* 2005 [cited March 14, 2006]; available from: http://www .ama-assn.org/ama/pub/category/14863.html.

Lo, B., McLeod, G. A., Saika, G. "Patient Attitudes to Discussing Life-Sustaining Treatment." *Archives of Internal Medicine* 1986;146(8): 1613–15.

Lockley, S. W., Cronin, J. W., Evans, E. E., et al. "Effect of Reducing Interns' Weekly Work Hours on Sleep and Attentional Failures." *New England Journal of Medicine* 2004;351(18):1829–37.

Lowenstein, J. "Where Have All the Giants Gone? Reconciling Medical Education and the Traditions of Patient Care with Limitations on Resident Work Hours." *Perspectives in Biology and Medicine* 2003;46(2):273–82.

Ludmerer, K. *Time to Heal: American Medical Education from the Turn of the Century to the Era of Managed Care.* New York: Oxford University Press, 1999.

Lynn, J. "Living Long in Fragile Health: The New Demographics Shape End of Life Care." *Hastings Center Report* 2005;Spec No:S14–18.

Lynn, J. "Perspectives on Care at the Close of Life. Serving Patients Who May Die Soon and Their Families: The Role of Hospice and Other Services." *Journal of the American Medical Association* 2001;285(7): 925–32.

Lynn, J. *Sick to Death and Not Going to Take It Anymore!* Berkeley: University of California Press, 2004.

Lynn, J., Harrold, J. *Handbook for Mortals: Guidance for People Facing Serious Illness.* New York: Oxford University Press, 1999.

MacLeod, R. D. "On Reflection: Doctors Learning to Care for People Who Are Dying." *Social Science and Medicine* 2001;52(11):1719–27.

Marik, P. E., Varon, J., Lisbon, A., et al. "Physicians' Own Preferences to the Limitation and Withdrawal of Life-Sustaining Therapy." *Resuscitation* 1999;42(3):197–201.

Marks, S. C., Jr., Bertman, S. L., Penney, J. C. "Human Anatomy: A Foundation for Education About Death and Dying in Medicine." *Clinical Anatomy* 1997;10(2):118–22.

Mast, K. R., Salama, M., Silverman, G. K., et al. "End-of-Life Content in Treatment Guidelines for Life-Limiting Diseases." *Journal of Palliative Medicine* 2004;7(6):754–73.

McCahill, L. E., Dunn, G. P., Mosenthal, A. C., et al. "Palliation as a Core Surgical Principle: Part 2." *Journal of the American College of Surgeons* 2004;199(2):321–34.

McCahill, L. E., Krouse, R. S., Chu, D. Z., et al. "Decision Making in Palliative Surgery." *Journal of the American College of Surgeons* 2002;195(3):411–22; discussion 422–23.

McCahill, L. E., Smith, D. D., Borneman, T., et al. "A Prospective Evaluation of Palliative Outcomes for Surgery of Advanced Malignancies." *Annals of Surgical Oncology* 2003;10(6):654–63.

McDonagh, J. R., Elliott, T. B., Engelberg, R. A., et al. "Family Satisfaction with Family Conferences About End-of-Life Care in the Intensive Care Unit: Increased Proportion of Family Speech Is Associated with Increased Satisfaction." *Critical Care Medicine* 2004;32(7):1484–88.

McDowell, J. "The Corpus and the Hare." *Modern Drug Discovery* 2000;3(8):77–80.

McManus, I. C., Keeling, A., Paice, E. "Stress, Burnout and Doctors' Attitudes to Work Are Determined by Personality and Learning Style: A Twelve Year Longitudinal Study of UK Medical Graduates." *BMC Medicine* 2004;2:29.

Meier, D. E., Back, A. L., Morrison, R. S. "The Inner Life of Physicians and Care of the Seriously Ill." *Journal of the American Medical Association* 2001;286(23):3007–14.

Meisel, A., Snyder, L., Quill, T. "Seven Legal Barriers to End-of-Life Care: Myths, Realities, and Grains of Truth." *Journal of the American Medical Association* 2000;284(19):2495–2501.

Meropol, N. J., Weinfurt, K. P., Burnett, C. B., et al. "Perceptions of Patients and Physicians Regarding Phase I Cancer Clinical Trials: Implications for Physician-Patient Communication." *Journal of Clinical Oncology* 2003;21(13):2589–96.

Metcalf, P., Huntington, R. *Celebrations of Death: The Anthropology of Mortuary Ritual.* 2nd Ed. Cambridge: Cambridge University Press, 1991.

Meyers, F. J., Linder, J. "Simultaneous Care: Disease Treatment and Palliative Care Throughout Illness." *Journal of Clinical Oncology* 2003;21(7):1412–15.

Miller, M. N., McGowen, K. R. "The Painful Truth: Physicians Are Not Invincible." *Southern Medical Journal* 2000;93(10):966–73.

Mims, C. *When We Die: The Science, Culture, and Rituals of Death.* New York: St. Martin's Press, 1998.

Molmenti, E. P., Dunn, G. P. "Transplantation and Palliative Care: The Convergence of Two Seemingly Opposite Realities." *Surgical Clinics of North America* 2005;85(2):373–82.

Morrison, R. S., Maroney-Galin, C., Kralovec, P. D., et al. "The Growth of Palliative Care Programs in United States Hospitals." *Journal of Palliative Medicine* 2005;8(6):1127–34.

Morrison, R. S., Meier, D. E. "Clinical Practice: Palliative Care." *New England Journal of Medicine* 2004;350(25):2582–90.

Morrison, R. S., Siu, A. L., Leipzig, R. M., et al. "The Hard Task of Improving the Quality of Care at the End of Life." *Archives of Internal Medicine* 2000;160(6):743–47.

Mukherjee, S. "A Precarious Exchange." *New England Journal of Medicine* 2004;351(18):1822–24.

Mullan, F. "Seasons of Survival: Reflections of a Physician with Cancer." *New England Journal of Medicine* 1985;313(4):270–73.

Muller, J. H. "Shades of Blue: The Negotiation of Limited Codes by Medical Residents." *Social Science and Medicine* 1992;34(8):885–98.

Murayama, K. M., Derossis, A. M., DaRosa, D. A., et al. "A Critical Evaluation of the Morbidity and Mortality Conference." *American Journal of Surgery* 2002;183(3):246–50.

National Comprehensive Cancer Network. "Palliative Care: Clinical Practice Guidelines in Oncology." *Journal of the National Comprehensive Cancer Network* 2003;1(3):394–420.

National Hospice and Palliative Care Organization. "NHPCO's 2004 Facts and Figures." 2004 [cited March 8, 2006]; available from: http://www.nhpco.org/files/public/Facts_Figures_for2004data.pdf.

Novack, D. H., Plumer, R., Smith, R. L., et al. "Changes in Physicians' Attitudes Toward Telling the Cancer Patient." *Journal of the American Medical Association* 1979;241(9):897–900.

Nuland, S. *How We Die: Reflections on Life's Final Chapter.* New York: Vintage, 1993.

Oken, D. "What to Tell Cancer Patients. A Study of Medical Attitudes." *Journal of the American Medical Association* 1961;175:1120–28.

Orlander, J. D., Barber, T. W., Fincke, B. G. "The Morbidity and Mortality Conference: The Delicate Nature of Learning from Error." *Academic Medicine* 2002;77(10):1001–6.

Orlander, J. D., Fincke, B. G. "Morbidity and Mortality Conference: A Survey of Academic Internal Medicine Departments." *Journal of General Internal Medicine* 2003;18(8):656–58.

Ornstein, C., Zarembo, A. "The UCLA Body Parts Scandal." *Los Angeles Times,* March 10, 2004.

Peters, A. S., Greenberger-Rosovsky, R., Crowder, C., et al. "Long-Term Outcomes of the New Pathway Program at Harvard Medical School: A Randomized Controlled Trial." *Academic Medicine* 2000;75(5):470–79.

Phipps, E., True, G., Harris, D., et al. "Approaching the End of Life: Attitudes, Preferences, and Behaviors of African-American and White Patients and Their Family Caregivers." *Journal of Clinical Oncology* 2003;21(3):549–54.

Pierluissi, E., Fischer, M. A., Campbell, A. R., et al. "Discussion of Medical Errors in Morbidity and Mortality Conferences." *Journal of the American Medical Association* 2003;290(21):2838–42.

Porter-Williamson, K., von Gunten, C. F., Garman, K., et al. "Improving Knowledge in Palliative Medicine with a Required Hospice Rotation for Third-Year Medical Students." *Academic Medicine* 2004;79(8):777–82.

Poses, R. M., Bekes, C., Winkler, R. L., et al. "Are Two (Inexperienced) Heads Better than One (Experienced) Head? Averaging House Officers' Prognostic Judgments for Critically Ill Patients." *Archives of Internal Medicine* 1990;150:1874–78.

Poulson, J. "Bitter Pills to Swallow." *New England Journal of Medicine* 1998;338(25):1844–46.

Prendergast, T. J., Luce, J. M. "Increasing Incidence of Withholding and Withdrawal of Life Support from the Critically Ill." *American Journal of Respiratory and Critical Care Medicine* 1997;155:15–20.

Quill, T. E. "Perspectives on Care at the Close of Life. Initiating End-of-Life Discussions with Seriously Ill Patients: Addressing the 'Elephant in the Room.' " *Journal of the American Medical Association* 2000;284(19): 2502–7.

Rabow, M. W., Hardie, G. E., Fair, J. M., et al. "End-of-Life Care Content in 50 Textbooks from Multiple Specialties." *Journal of the American Medical Association* 2000;283(6):771–78.

Rappaport, W., Prevel, C., Witzke, D., et al. "Education About Death and

Dying During Surgical Residency." *American Journal of Surgery* 1991;161(6):690–92.

Rappaport, W., Witzke, D. "Education About Death and Dying During the Clinical Years of Medical School." *Surgery* 1993;113(2):163–65.

Ratanawongsa, N., Teherani, A., Hauer, K. E. "Third-Year Medical Students' Experiences with Dying Patients During the Internal Medicine Clerkship: A Qualitative Study of the Informal Curriculum." *Academic Medicine* 2005;80(7):641–47.

Razavi, D., Merckaert, I., Marchal, S., et al. "How to Optimize Physicians' Communication Skills in Cancer Care: Results of a Randomized Study Assessing the Usefulness of Posttraining Consolidation Workshops." *Journal of Clinical Oncology* 2003;21(16):3141–49.

Redinbaugh, E. M., Sullivan, A. M., Block, S. D., et al. "Doctors' Emotional Reactions to Recent Death of a Patient: Cross Sectional Study of Hospital Doctors." *British Medical Journal* 2003;327(7408):185.

Reifler, D. R. " 'I Actually Don't Mind the Bone Saw': Narratives of Gross Anatomy." *Literature and Medicine* 1996;15(2):183–99.

Rhodes-Kropf, J., Carmody, S. S., Seltzer, D., et al. " 'This Is Just Too Awful; I Just Can't Believe I Experienced That.' Medical Students' Reactions to Their 'Most Memorable' Patient Death." *Academic Medicine* 2005;80(7):634–40.

Richardson, R. *Death, Dissection and the Destitute.* Chicago: University of Chicago Press, 2000.

Risucci, D. A., Sullivan, T., DiRusso, S., et al. "Assessing Educational Validity of the Morbidity and Mortality Conference: A Pilot Study." *Current Surgery* 2003;60(2):204–9.

Roach, M. *Stiff: The Curious Lives of Human Cadavers.* New York: W. W. Norton, 2003.

Roberson, D. W., Sachdeva, A., Healy, G. B. "Morbidity and Mortality Conference: Both Ahead of Its Time and Behind the Times. Surgical M + M and Patient Safety 2005" [cited March 15, 2006]; available from: http://www.facs.org/education/surgical-m-and-m/featured_article.html.

Robins, L. S., White, C. B., Fantone, J. C. "The Difficulty of Sustaining Curricular Reforms: A Study of 'Drift' at One School." *Academic Medicine* 2000;75(8):801–5.

Rothman, E. L. *White Coat: Becoming a Doctor at Harvard Medical School.* New York: William Morrow, 1999.

Rousseau, P. "Aggressive Treatment in the Terminally Ill: Right or Wrong?" *Journal of Palliative Medicine* 2002;5(5):657–58.

Satel, S. "Doctors Behind Bars: Treating Pain Is Now Risky Business." 2004 [cited March 24, 2006]; available from: http://www.nytimes.com/2004/10/19/health/policy/19essa.html?ex=1143349200&en=c332077cf483322b&ei=5070.

Schwartz, C. E., Goulet, J. L., Gorski, V., et al. "Medical Residents' Perceptions of End-of-Life Care Training in a Large Urban Teaching Hospital." *Journal of Palliative Medicine* 2003;6(1):37–44.

Selzer, R. *Raising the Dead: A Doctor's Encounter with His Own Mortality.* New York: Penguin, 1993.

Shafer, A. "Art Annotations: Fildes, Sir Luke—The Doctor." Literature, Arts, and Medicine Database 2000 (revised 2002) [cited May 5, 2006]; available from: http://endeavor.med.nyu.edu/lit-med/lit-med-db/web docs/webart/fildes50-art-.html.

Sharkey, F. *A Parting Gift.* New York: Bantam, 1982.

Solomon, M. Z., O'Donnell, L., Jennings, B., et al. "Decisions Near the End of Life: Professional Views on Life-Sustaining Treatments." *American Journal of Public Health* 1993;83(1):14–23.

Spiro, H. M. "The Silence of Words—Some Thoughts on the Pernkopf Atlas." *Wien Klin Wochenschr* 1998;110(4–5):183–84.

Spiro, H. M., Mandell, H. N. "When Doctors Get Sick." *Annals of Internal Medicine* 1998;128(2):152–54.

Steinhauser, K. E., Christakis, N.A., Clipp, E.C., et al. "Factors Considered Important at the End of Life by Patients, Family, Physicians, and Other Care Providers." *Journal of the American Medical Association* 2000;284(19):2476–82.

Steinhauser, K. E., Clipp, E. C., McNeilly, M., et al. "In Search of a Good Death: Observations of Patients, Families, and Providers." *Annals of Internal Medicine* 2000;132(10):825–32.

Stevens, L., Cook, D., Guyatt, G., et al. "Education, Ethics, and End-of-Life Decisions in the Intensive Care Unit." *Critical Care Medicine* 2002;30(2):290–96.

Sullivan, A. M., Lakoma, M. D., Block, S. D. "The Status of Medical Education in End-of-Life Care: A National Report." *Journal of General Internal Medicine* 2003;18(9):685–95.

Sullivan, A. M., Warren, A. G., Lakoma, M. D., et al. "End-of-Life Care in the Curriculum: A National Study of Medical Education Deans." *Academic Medicine* 2004;79(8):760–68.

SUPPORT Principal Investigators. "A Controlled Trial to Improve Care for Seriously Ill Hospitalized Patients. The Study to Understand Prognoses and Preferences for Outcomes and Risks of Treatments (SUPPORT). The

SUPPORT Principal Investigators." *Journal of the American Medical Association* 1995;274(20):1591–98.

Surgeons Palliative Care Workgroup. "Office of Promoting Excellence in End-of-Life Care: Surgeons Palliative Care Workgroup Report from the Field." *Journal of the American College of Surgeons* 2003;197(4):661–86.

Terkel, S. "Dr. John Barrett." In: *Will the Circle Be Unbroken? Reflections on Death, Rebirth, and Hunger for a Faith.* New York: Ballantine, 2001: 29–38.

Terkel, S. "Dr. Sharon Sandell." In: *Will the Circle Be Unbroken? Reflections on Death, Rebirth, and Hunger for a Faith.* New York: Ballantine, 2001: 24–28.

Tolstoy, L. *The Death of Ivan Ilyich.* New York: Bantam, 1981.

Tulsky, J. A., Chesney, M. A., Lo, B. "How Do Medical Residents Discuss Resuscitation with Patients?" *Journal of General Internal Medicine* 1995;10(8):436–42.

Tulsky, J. A., Chesney, M. A., Lo, B. "See One, Do One, Teach One? House Staff Experience Discussing Do-Not-Resuscitate Orders." *Archives of Internal Medicine* 1996;156(12):1285–89.

Tulsky, J. A., Fischer, G. S., Rose, M. R., et al. "Opening the Black Box: How Do Physicians Communicate About Advance Directives?" *Annals of Internal Medicine* 1998;129(6):441–49.

Tward, A. D., Patterson, H. A. "From Grave Robbing to Gifting: Cadaver Supply in the United States." *Journal of the American Medical Association* 2002;287(9):1183.

Veldenz, H. C., Dovgan, P. S., Schinco, M. S., et al. "Morbidity and Mortality Conference: Enhancing Delivery of Surgery Residency Curricula." *Current Surgery* 2001;58(6):580–82.

Ventres, W., Nichter, M., Reed, R., et al. "Do-Not-Resuscitate Discussions: A Qualitative Analysis." *Family Practice Research Journal* 1992;12(2):157–69.

Verghese, A. "The Calling." *New England Journal of Medicine* 2005;352(18):1844–47.

Verghese, A. "The Physician as Storyteller." *Annals of Internal Medicine* 2001;135(11):1012–17.

Von Gunten, C. F., Ferris, F. D., Emanuel, L. L. "The Patient-Physician Relationship. Ensuring Competency in End-of-Life Care: Communication and Relational Skills." *Journal of the American Medical Association* 2000;284(23):3051–57.

Walter, T. "Historical and Cultural Variants on the Good Death." *British Medical Journal* 2003;327(7408):218–20.

Webb, M. *The Good Death: The New American Search to Reshape the End of Life*. New York: Bantam, 1997.

Weinstein, A. *A Scream Goes Through the House: What Literature Teaches Us About Life*. New York: Random House, 2003.

Weiss, S. C., Emanuel, L. L., Fairclough, D. L., et al. "Understanding the Experience of Pain in Terminally Ill Patients." *Lancet* 2001;357(9265): 1311–15.

Weissman, D. E., Block, S. D. "ACGME Requirements for End-of-Life Training in Selected Residency and Fellowship Programs: A Status Report." *Academic Medicine* 2002;77(4):299–304.

Weissman, D. E., Block, S. D., Blank, L., et al. "Recommendations for Incorporating Palliative Care Education into the Acute Care Hospital Setting." *Academic Medicine* 1999;74(8):871–77.

Wenrich, M. D., Curtis, J. R., Shannon, S. E., et al. "Communicating with Dying Patients Within the Spectrum of Medical Care from Terminal Diagnosis to Death." *Archives of Internal Medicine* 2001;161(6):868–74.

Whippen, D. A., Canellos, G. P. "Burnout Syndrome in the Practice of Oncology: Results of a Random Survey of 1,000 Oncologists." *Journal of Clinical Oncology* 1991;9(10):1916–20.

Williams, C. M., Wilson, C. C., Olsen, C. H. "Dying, Death, and Medical Education: Student Voices." *Journal of Palliative Medicine* 2005;8(2):372–81.

World Health Organization. "WHO Definition of Palliative Care." [cited March 8, 2006]; available from: http://www.who.int/cancer/palliative/definition/en/.

Yun, Y. H., Lee, C. G., Kim, S. Y., et al. "The Attitudes of Cancer Patients and Their Families Toward the Disclosure of Terminal Illness." *Journal of Clinical Oncology* 2004;22(2):307–14.

Zuger, A. "Dissatisfaction with Medical Practice." *New England Journal of Medicine* 2004;350(1):69–75.

Zuger, A. "Doctors Learn How to Say What No One Wants to Hear." *New York Times*, January 10, 2006, Sect. F1.